THE
DETOURS

Published by Deeds Publishing
Marietta, GA
www.deedspublishing.com

Printed in the United States of America

Cover design by Mark Babcock

Library of Congress Cataloging-in-Publications Data is available upon request.

ISBN 978-1-937565-27-5

Books are available in quantity for promotional or premium use. For information, write Deeds Publishing, PO Box 682212, Marietta, GA 30068 or info@deedspublishing.com.

First Edition, 2012

10 9 8 7 6 5 4 3 2 1

THE DETOURS

{*neil ligon*}

This book is dedicated to Em Ligon, the strongest mother I can imagine, since without her endless support and understanding, I would not be here today, and Carrie Lofstrom, who fills my days with love and hope, and whose encouragement made sure that a story stored on scraps of paper and in the recesses of a broken brain would find its way onto the pages that follow.

Ten percent of the proceeds earned from the sale of this book by Deeds Publishing and Neil Ligon will be donated to the Emory Chapter of the Brain Injury Association of Georgia and the Brain Injury Peer Visitor Association, both terrific organizations that provide invaluable support for brain injured individuals, their families and caretakers.

{introduction}

An accident stole from me what was mine. It took what I had been promised.

I knew this by the beginning of 2005. But I understood almost nothing else, and I appeared to be incapable of learning.

Was it an accident or punishment for past mistakes? What exactly had been stolen and how had I ever come to possess it? What had I been promised?

I feared the questions, so I tried to stop asking them. I stagnated. I survived. I obsessed: over the theft, what was missing, what path my life should have followed. The present vanished far more quickly than the past reappeared. For more than five years, I bounced from voice to voice, begging affirmation for my present self—surviving until the next day, when I hoped the necessary epiphanies would appear. But time and again I failed to assign sufficient meaning to a life that I was living half-heartedly and the questions remained.

I told myself there wasn't time to worry about such trivialities. I had a document review deadline next week, friends to meet for beers next Thursday, bills to worry about, a softball game tomorrow night…until, without warning, there weren't any documents in my queue at work, my friends began to leave town, the bills became manageable, and the intramural successes couldn't fill the void.

It was then that I quit my job to write this book. It wasn't that this choice was forced on me. I knew the workflow would resume, new friendships would arise, recent plays made during softball games would leave me with a sense of accomplishment for days at a time. But it wasn't enough. I walked away of my own volition from the life I had come to know to write my story, to address the questions I couldn't stop asking.

I need these stories to mean something to me. Even as I sit down to complete the monumental task of reassembling them, I know they may never be as valuable to me as the time I lost collecting them. But that is a risk I am finally willing to take.

Because of the possibility of misstatement, the product of a message whispered down a line, each telling distorting the story in some way and misconstruing certain specific details, names have been changed to avoid any potential prejudice that would be suffered by those individuals whose only mistake was coming into contact with a confused, broken boy.

I am trapped by a past that others have built for me and that I cannot fully comprehend. It is time for me to try to understand it.

I didn't die. That means something to me. The life that followed needs to, too.

the
blocked
path

{chapter 1}

It began as someone else's story dictated to me, though I wanted parts of it to be mine. Like a student fresh out of school, I wanted the carefree innocence to persist. I wanted the past to weave seamlessly into my present, a tale of success that I could deliver on cue with a look. I couldn't have known this vision was to disappear in a second and be replaced by what I now hold: a mangled mass of unintelligible loss.

A rapacious universe has taken what it once freely gave me and left me no token by which to remember this time. The hazy memories—formerly shadows dancing in the background, snippets of sound or random images representing seconds of hour-long events—in an increasingly opaque narrative told by others, became fewer and fewer, until, at last, the absence was all that remained.

According to my girlfriend Amy, when I started the tedious trip, it was a normal Louisiana day, hot and humid, but otherwise clear. No flickering images remain in my head that would tell another tale, but another one soon unfolded. As the trip continued, the sky darkened, and the standard afternoon showers began. My automobile sliced through the precipitation, continuing along the dampening pavement with me inside, unconcerned. The driving rain pounded my windshield but, unlike the storms to which I was accustomed, this one continued to grow stronger as I continued across Alabama, still only three hours into my trip. Visibility barely extended a few yards beyond the hood of my car, but I soldiered on in my quest to get to Aiken, squinting to see the reflective paint of the highway's lines, the car's cruise control maintaining my speed while I focused exclusively on navigating the vehicle.

The vehicle protected me from the elements, and its automated systems seemed to further promise the assistance necessary to make it through the storm. But the guidance was misleading, and a stretch of I-65 ninety miles north of Mobile soon wrested away my autonomy and rendered me powerless. Without warning, the car's wheels suddenly lost their grip on the road, and the vehicle slid across the slick roadway. During those final moments, I struggled to maintain my intended path, but attempts to correct for the loss of traction proved ineffective. The car approached the pavement's edge with me still helplessly fighting a steering column that no longer offered me even the illusion of control. Everything was about to change.

The police report and its accompanying illustrations described the skid but omitted the unadulterated fear, since my emotional state was irrelevant to the outcome. The Explorer, which had begun its insolence at over 70 mph, tore down the hill running parallel to the road at an unmeasured pace, but one close to its prior speed. The wheels left the ground and the vehicle's energy dissipated, performing its final cartwheels that threw my wallet and my memories free of the vehicle, leveling a roadside sign before vaulting a stream and finally coming to rest on its side with me inside, suspended by my seat belt. Glass from the shattered driver's side window, a result of either impact with my head during the rolls or the pressure transferred from the frame as the car flipped, was scattered everywhere around me. My trip had concluded with a detour and, due to the weather, my new destination at the bottom of this hill was next to an empty stretch of I-65. No one rushed to my rescue.

A couple on their way to a wedding eventually drove by, and, out of the corner of his eye, the driver was able to make out what he believed to be the outline of a car on the side of the road, lying in a ditch in front of the roadside trees. The couple drove on for a few more moments before he decided to investigate. He impulsively pulled their car onto the shoulder and returned in reverse to where he believed he had seen the car. Upon their arrival, the couple confirmed that it was indeed an overturned vehicle, and they descended the hill to inspect it.

When they arrived at the base of the hill, the couple was greeted by a softly moaning person hanging by his seat belt and they called 911 to report it. The engine was cold, indicating the car had been there for a while. She held my hand while they awaited the medical rescue team and promised me everything would be all right. We would not attempt dialogue for four more years, when I began my final attempt to understand.

The police, firemen and medical team soon made it to me, and the whirring of the Jaws of Life and the screeching of surrendering metal provided the change music, as they dislodged me from the automobile and rushed me to the next scene at the nearest hospital.

My wallet, stuffed too full of old receipts to comfortably sit on, had previously rested on my front seat, and it contained my driver's license, a South Carolina license listing Mom's address as my permanent address. A woman who'd been driving by, stopped when she saw the police lights and, using the driver's license address in the wallet she saw next to the road, she obtained a phone number through information and called it. It was an inversion of the process I had always feared. Mom's previous heart attacks and her blood pressure spikes had kept me up at night plenty of times throughout law school and had left me terrified of the random unknown phone call. Now strangers were delivering unwanted news, but not to me. Mom was to join me in the world of the unknown.

{chapter 2}

Why was Mom standing in her house on August 30, 2004, hearing news of an event that shouldn't have happened? Everything had already been scripted, and it was supposed to end well. Any doubt of where I was going to arrive had been erased by a mixture of hard work and fortuitous breaks. The journey had begun long before I slid behind the wheel that day.

During May of that year, I had participated in a ceremony that marked the end of my days as an academic—I was officially a law school graduate. My work ethic had been but a reflection of the consequences my laziness would leave me to face, so to call my final year at Tulane an academic period was to strain language to the breaking point. I intended the days to be just one final party before the work grind began. But the years preceding this celebration hadn't been as comfortable.

My first year in law school, I had worked diligently to build stability. The day after I moved into my house in New Orleans to begin law school, I met an attractive, intelligent woman who lived next door, and our exchanges became more than platonic soon after our first meeting. As the first semester of school started and other friendships were only just beginning to form, we were already spending hours together, sharing the uncertainty of new law students. I typed and retyped my notes and memorized highlighted passages from my law books and the case names that were important, and we learned with one another. She laughed at my jokes while we studied, and often even our breaks from the information deluge were together. I impulsively proposed six weeks later, and she accepted, guaranteeing certainty in a time plagued by doubt.

This stability ended when the relationship dissolved in short order, a victim of too much stress, too little due diligence prior to our commitment to one another, and our youth, and I turned to school for comfort. My friendships were still limited in number and quality, so I had no other outlet for my energies. The threatening solitude made the books my friends, and my grades reflected this, placing me in the top five percent of my class, after the defections of some elite students to more highly regarded schools, a ranking that secured my place on law review.

During the second year of my studies, my life became more balanced. Friendships formed at the nearby gym playing pick-up basketball and on the intramural athletic fields playing softball grew into accepting social groups. My newly discovered scholastic aptitudes were rewarded with multiple interviews and quite a few offers of summer employment at prestigious law firms in Atlanta, one of which I accepted. When the school year ended in May, I headed to Atlanta for the summer to pursue professional success at Irwin Myers.

That summer found me fighting to maintain my place in the elite, this time in an attempt to gain a position of permanent employment. All of the other interns were members of the upper tier at their elite schools as well, and when I weighed the competition, I saw my intellectual inferiority. I made sure to stay a little longer than everyone else while I refined my memos detailing the law I was assigned to research, and I hoped my efforts had not gone unnoticed. August arrived and with it the end of my internship, and I left for New Orleans to complete my final year of school. A few people at Irwin Myers who were familiar with the process assured me that the firm would formally make me an offer soon.

When I returned to school, buoyed by the knowledge that an almost six figure salary awaited me in Atlanta, the entirety of my third year of law school degenerated into an exercise in indulgence. Beer and football dominated my weekends and much of my week as well, and I spent more of my time running up and down Tulane's basketball courts heaving up fifteen-foot jump shots with reckless abandon than I did attending my classes and contemplating legal theory. I was already coasting my way through my final year of law school in anticipation of the firm's offer of employment, and when I began the second semester of my third year of school with that formal offer in hand, my vacation officially commenced.

As intemperate as the first semester of my final year had been, it was the second semester that marked the apex of my blossoming ego, which rested comfortably on the illusory laurels that a letter grade so aptly conveys. I had finally become comfortable, maybe even too comfortable, in my own skin.

Football season was over, so without this televised distraction, my attentions turned to a variety of other extracurricular activities, including intramural softball, where I hit tenth and played catcher on a team stacked with former high school ball players and a few former Division I talents; intramural basketball, where I was an adequate last-guy-off-the-bench thanks to my six-foot-two stature; drinking to excess, a frequent hobby of mine and others in the city of New Orleans; and chasing women, where I remained woefully inept but benefitted from a dearth of viable alternatives. I allegedly picked up the ego-massaging nickname "the hot TA," bestowed on me by a group of first year students in the Legal Research and Writing section for which I was one of the teaching assistants. Although this title was conveyed to me by Amy, a first year student with whom I began a relationship after my TA duties were complete, I never questioned the veracity of her claim and clung to it stubbornly, because the label fit perfectly with how I wanted to be perceived.

Reality interjected itself periodically. Todd, the associate at Irwin Myers with whom I had become friends during my internship, cautioned me to enjoy myself but to make sure I graduated. Although my spotty attendance in class gave rise to fears of failure, the combination of a well-chosen class schedule and a few weeks of hard work was enough to ensure passing marks. The festivities on graduation day—May 22, 2004—included me, and I still graduated with Honors, though I was one of the few members of law review to not graduate with High Honors.

My extended family, a small but geographically scattered group, came in from around the country to celebrate. My brother Colin arrived from the North, where he was graduating from Princeton the following week, and the Midwestern contingent, encompassing members of both sides of my family joined as well: my cousin Jason from my dad's side of the family and his wife Alison arrived from Kentucky and my Uncle Felix from my mom's side and his wife Mary came in from Chicago. Mom came from the East, making the trek from Aiken, South Carolina, a town a few miles across the border from Augusta, Georgia. I did my best to coordinate the logistics of procuring tickets to everything for all who had come down, and Mom planned our evening meals and covered the costs.

The inconsistent focus that marked my third year in law school, though taken to the extreme during those final months, was not wholly new, and my rollercoaster career in school had not left Mom much time for peace—my lackluster effort as an undergraduate student at The University of Virginia during my first year there had resulted in academic probation. My study habits while there, fueled by No-Doze and Mountain Dew, consisted of answering a semester of indolence with a few well-timed all-nighters to crank out papers, or a series of all-nighters to finish the necessary reading I had yet to complete for classes where my attendance narrowly crested the sixty percent mark.

Now that I had my law school diploma in hand and a job awaiting me, she could finally exhale. I felt so proud, looking around at my family, knowing my graduation was an accomplishment, and I enjoyed every second, believing this would sufficiently label me successful for life. My voice was as loud as ever as I asserted opinion after opinion with a self-assuredness born of naivety and a complete disregard for my potential ignorance of the moment's subject matter. I thought I had already been marked by life as one of the chosen and that it was only a matter of time before I was officially anointed as a successful adult.

After the final celebrations in New Orleans, I returned to Atlanta and spent the next two months studying to pass the Georgia Bar Exam, which I believed was the last remaining hurdle before I could begin my successful legal career. The summer following my graduation was funded by a signing bonus from my new firm, which guaranteed I could cover rent. One of my roommates from law school, Kevin Butler, lived with me that summer, and we both attended a bar preparation class held at Emory University. Perhaps my earlier study habits continued, as he claimed, and PlayStation continued to dominate my afternoons, but I do not remember much of this time and cannot say for sure. Regardless, the practice tests soon indicated that my preparation would not be sufficient, and, as my bar class wound down, I began spending time at the office of my future employer, cramming as much information as I possibly could into my head.

I still found time to play on the firm's intramural teams and socialize with the younger summer interns, but as the exam date drew nearer, I eliminated all outside distractions for a final cramming period. The specter of failure again began to haunt me, and the days of fear-motivated studying ended with an unshakable sense of dread. I sought reassurance from my future coworker Todd. What would happen if I did not pass?

"You will just have to retake it," he told me.

It was comforting that my job wasn't on the line.

"But none of our lawyers have ever failed the Georgia bar," he continued.

I spent the remaining days reminding myself that failure had no true repercussions, though I already knew that my reputation would be difficult to alter once it was established, and that this was not a blight I wanted on my resume at the beginning of my career.

The big event finally arrived. Kevin and I rented a hotel room near the test site, and he drove us to the exam, held in the enormous auditorium of the Georgia International Convention Center. The exam began on my birthday, July 27, and the first part tested knowledge of Georgia state law with a series of essay questions to be answered within the allotted time.

The first question of the morning session was right in my wheelhouse, and my pen flew across the paper as if it had a mind of its own—months of knowledge pouring onto the page, my ink capturing every possibly related law I could remember to support my answer. Amidst a room of agitated, panicked people, I sat smiling, flooding the page with information.

Suddenly, I noticed that my verbosity had left me with less than a page to answer the third part of a three-part question. Panic washed over me, and my pen slowed, as I began writing in 4-point font. I squeezed as much information as I could fit into the remaining space in the booklet, but as our time ran down and my margins overflowed with barely legible phrases, I knew it was insufficient. When test administrators briefly released us for our lunch break between sections, Kevin and I unsteadily moved toward the exit to stretch our legs. I was inconsolably upset.

"I need to go home. I've already failed," I grieved.

"I have to stay here and finish. I don't know how you are going to get home," Kevin wearily responded.

Without options, I resumed my test taking after lunch, and when the day was done, I walked to the car with Kevin, completely shell-shocked. We headed back to the hotel for the evening, where I attempted to cram whatever additional information my saturated brain could hold. The next morning, we were back at our auditorium for the national multiple choice portion of the exam. The information I had learned the night before was long gone by the time I took my seat, but I didn't really care anymore. My fate was already sealed. After a day of nerve-wracking decisions hurriedly made without hope, time was suddenly announced, and we filed out with the rest of the defeated.

Our first stop was at a nearby bar, with one of our fellow Tulane graduates, to wearily celebrate the completion of the test with fried bar food and a token beer that we grudgingly forced down.

"Happy birthday, man. At least that shit is finally over, and we're drinking beer. I'm sure you did fine."

Even as we talked, I was already considering how I was going to deal with the bitter reality that I had not done fine. I had failed and would have to retake it. With that fact weighing heavily on me, there was still some form of relief, as the ordeal was temporarily over, and by the third sip of beer, I quit worrying about my future problems and began to calm down.

Amy, the first year law student from my legal research and writing class, and I had spent the summer dating long distance. I left her a message that night to let her know I had survived. Then I wandered out the door for the nearby bars. It was time to relax until October, when I was sure to be crowned a success regardless of my bar results.

After that night, the summer began in earnest, since I had no additional responsibilities until I was to begin my job two months later. Mom purchased a frequent flier ticket for me for my birthday so I could go visit my friend from Aiken and UVA, Shawn Carlson, who was a Navy helicopter pilot then stationed in Honolulu. I arranged to visit another friend from

UVA, Karen, who lived in Baltimore while she attended Johns Hopkins getting her Ph.D. in History. The days ahead began to fill with the kind of obligations that many dreamed of having.

A week after we finished taking the bar exam, Kevin moved out and on with his life and headed down to Mobile for his judicial clerkship. After a couple weeks of lying around being useless, I knew I needed to find a way to better occupy my time, since I too frequently found myself standing in Circuit City with my hands full of movies, drawing down the few remaining summer dollars in my bank account.

"You could always come down and visit me," Amy suggested one evening during our nightly phone conversation. Spending a weekend in New Orleans with my girlfriend was far more enticing than another week in Atlanta, no matter what new releases were due out, so I packed a bag, jumped in my car, and headed for her place. With no pressing plans in Atlanta, my stay predictably extended into the following week. That Monday evening, my phone rang with an 803 number I didn't recognize. It was one of Mom's friends.

"Neil, I wanted to let you know that your mom is really sick with pneumonia, and we had to take her to the emergency room Saturday night," she told me. "The doctor put her on a bunch of medication, and she is at home resting. Though she is responding well to the treatment, she is still feeling pretty terrible."

By the time the conversation concluded, I knew I needed to go see how Mom was doing. It was time to leave New Orleans anyway, so I passed the information along to Amy.

"My mom is sick, and I need to go check on her. I'll leave tomorrow morning after you get back from class," I explained to her. "I don't know if I will make it down again before I start work, but you can come up and visit me anytime you want; just give me a couple of days notice to make sure I'm in town, and I will grab Braves tickets or something else like that."

{the blocked path}

The next day, when she returned from class around eleven-thirty, I kissed her goodbye and headed for Aiken, South Carolina. It was a boring interstate drive I wished to put behind me. My late start was of no consequence to me; frequent trips home during law school established my familiarity with this stretch of road, which held no mysteries. I pulled the car door shut, waved a final goodbye, and departed for the interstate to begin my trip through Louisiana on I-10, heading toward I-65 and its monotonous journey across flat, rural Alabama. Even with the stretches of I-85 and I-20 that followed my time in Alabama, since I drove fast, I always planned on completing the drive inside of nine hours.

The phone call would beat me home, and I would not finish this trip for over two months.

{chapter 3}

"I'm really sorry to call you with such bad news, but I thought you would want to know," the voice began. "I found this wallet on the highway. I think it belongs to the person who is in the car at the bottom of this hill. I asked one of the police officers, and he told me they are taking the person to Evergreen Medical Center. You can call the hospital, and they will have more information."

Anticipating the arrival of her son, my mom was delivered this wilted bouquet of words in his place. Mom stood in her kitchen, horrified and frozen, listening to what the woman told her. The vocal paralysis did not last long.

"Is he ok? What's going on? Can you see him?"

"I don't know. They said the hospital will have more information."

Still sick with pneumonia, adrenaline coursing through her veins even as normal levels of oxygen did not, Mom frantically called the hospital and left her contact information so they could call her once I arrived and they began their diagnosis. She then immediately called Amy.

"Amy, this is Em," Mom intoned from her empty kitchen in Aiken, her despondency remaining veiled by a wall of shock and disbelief. "Neil has been in an accident. I don't have a lot of information right now, but I know that it's not good. I'm still really sick, and if they know he's not going to make it, I'm not going to rush down there."

The horror traveled through the phone and infected a new location. Amy's roommate jumped into the driver's seat, Amy crawled into the passenger seat, and they raced toward Evergreen Hospital. Along the way, she called her friend and former law school attendee Andrea, who had days before returned from her honeymoon; her new husband was one of my friends from law school.

Weeks before this moment, I had thrown back Bombay Sapphire and tonics at their wedding until my body purged the last of a bad idea out of my system and over the country club railing in front of disgusted fellow guests. They were not to be free of the embarrassment that I could will onto those around me yet, but the incidents which followed were no longer to be grounded in my immaturity. Andrea picked up and responded to the unexpected call by telling Amy that she would pick up her husband and my law school roommate Kevin, who was also living in Mobile, and meet her at the hospital.

Mom, waiting in Aiken, finally received a call from an emergency room doctor at Evergreen Hospital with the unpleasant news. The prognosis was no more reassuring than the initial message. The doctor informed her that the likelihood of my survival stood at around ten to fifteen percent.

"We're getting him ready to move, and then we will be taking him to the trauma hospital in Mobile. We cannot medevac him there by helicopter because we can't take the helicopter up in this weather, so we are going to have to put him in an ambulance."

He was describing chaos to a woman in need of certainty—certainty that my grandmother's words, spoken in a church filled with pain with my father's ashes resting in an urn at the front, would not haunt her, too.

"No mother should outlive her son," she had whispered.

Their children had looked so healthy.

The doctor could promise Mom nothing, but he offered what he could.

"I know this is a lot to take in, but he has a couple of very important things going for him. He is young, and we will soon have him at the University of South Alabama Medical Center, where he will have access to state of the art equipment and people who are accustomed to dealing with injuries like this."

Mom's boyfriend at the time was a physician at an Army base in Columbia, and he consoled her with the fact that the game changed in its entirety upon arrival at a trauma hospital, and the initial prognosis would be completely re-evaluated once I arrived in Mobile.

Mom's next call informed Amy of the change in location and the low likelihood of survival, and Amy passed the information along to Andrea from the passenger seat of her roommate's speeding car. Andrea, as promised, gathered her husband and Kevin, and they made it to the hospital before the ambulance. Upon their arrival, they were assigned a private waiting room that they filled with their agitated expansion while awaiting my arrival. At last I commanded the audience for which I had always longed, because I was finally special. I was not present.

Amy entered the hospital two minutes before the ambulance, and joined the law school group that sat waiting with no idea of what to expect. At last, the ambulance arrived, and my body was immediately whisked away for the doctors to begin working again. My friends were left confined to their waiting room, where I was not present to hear their conversation, and time muted it for everyone else. Once I was moved to the ICU, a doctor finally emerged with the prognosis.

"He has had a severe traumatic brain injury," he explained to the waiting group. "I'm not sure how he is going to come out of this or what kind of quality of life he will have."

"We can deal with the effects later," Amy snapped at him. "I need to know what is happening now. I need to be able to call his mother and tell her that her son is not going to die."

A puzzled look momentarily flashed on his face before he answered her quickly.

"He will live."

After the doctor's pronouncement, he exited the room, and a nurse entered and informed my visitors that they could see me, but only two at a time. Amy first called Mom to let her know that they now expected me to live. But the relief at this good news was short-lived. As the viewing began, she took her rightful spot as first mourner, unaware of her title and the quantity of bad news that awaited her entrance into that room over the following months. In this moment, she was not alone—my former roommate and fellow Georgia Bar student Kevin joined her. Expecting the most horrific sight, a strangely different one greeted them.

I lay flat on my back in the bed, and aside from a few cuts, I looked similar to the boy who had departed Amy's house less than twelve hours before. Yet the machines that surrounded me told a different tale. A ventilator forcefully breathed into the apparatus which emerged from my mouth, and assorted tubes ran from my arms to accompanying IV bags. I was barely alive, and everything around me indicated that the unseen problems were daunting. There were no default responses available, no reflexive verbal crutches to soothe the psyches of the witnesses. Instead, Amy absorbed the entire blow of what she saw and staggered back a bit, as Kevin put his arm around her to catch and console her. The good news of a few moments ago disappeared into the ether as reality slowly came into focus.

Back in Aiken, after the call from the innocent bystander, the news of my accident spread rapidly. A group of Mom's friends snapped into action and convened in her kitchen. The committee, a diverse body of her friends, which included a physician, began implementing executive decisions. Dr. Griffen took Mom's vitals, and after examining her, determined that though she was still not fully recovered from pneumonia, she was fit to travel.

But she couldn't travel alone, they agreed.

"I will go with her," her friend Kim forcefully asserted, and found no protests from the remaining members of the group.

The other parties were on their phones, bombarding airlines with a deluge of flight requests, trying to find the first plane out. They claimed two seats on the six o'clock flight the next morning for Mom and Kim.

In the midst of all the deliberate planning around her, Mom still could not come to grips with what was happening.

"I won't let God take him from me," she hissed between clinched teeth as the trip details finalized. But she didn't get to choose her losses, and her plans did not matter. She wouldn't even be present in Alabama for another twelve hours.

When her flight from Augusta did touch down early the next morning, Amy sent my old roommate Kevin to pick up Mom and Kim and shuttle them back to the hospital. By the time Mom arrived, my previous evening's appearance had worsened.

My head was so swollen that I was not readily identifiable. My neck was the size of a NFL linebacker's. I had two black eyes that were likely caused by my face bouncing off the airbag and into less forgiving interior fixtures during the car's roll. The intake form detailed all of the damage. The black eyes were the outward manifestation of a fractured left eye orbital, an ordinarily resilient structure that had not suffered the trauma as quietly as one would have hoped, and fractures to the walls of the right maxillary sinus. Additionally, though my tongue remained attached, it clung to my mouth by a thread, as I had almost bitten it off when my teeth rattled shut during the accident. Thus, my mouth contained a black, fetid mass that left no room for anything else to be visible.

The news was not all bad, though the optimists who delivered anything else seemed myopic. One of my doctors happily explained to Mom that my nose was not broken, which was quite fortuitous in his mind in light of the other fractures.

His announcement was not received with the same joy with which it was delivered.

My friend Shawn's parents arrived early that afternoon with my brother, Colin, who they had picked up in Charleston, where he was completing the summer session at Medical College of South Carolina. He joined the group standing in the room viewing my battered body and initially remained only for a few minutes before exiting to regain his composure. Mom's boyfriend arrived at the hospital a few hours later, and he asked to see my x-rays. After receiving permission, he took Colin with him to survey the medical situation, in a successful attempt to move the scene unfolding before my brother from the personal back to the clinical.

The hospital was a trauma hospital, and my state of being reflected as much. Any optimism would forever be dampened by the title of my accommodations. Nonetheless, within the first couple of days, I began to stabilize as the medical staff rushed about the ward. Some signs that a recovery had begun to take hold appeared even in those early days, and my visitors' hope was no longer an unfounded delusion. But all progress moved incrementally. Concerned that I could not effectively communicate potential issues with breathing, the doctors kept the intubation tube in place even when I was stable enough to no longer require life support.

Despite the life-saving capabilities of this device, all parties involved were aware of how unpleasant its presence was for me, due to my frequent struggles to remove it. To remedy the problem, the hospital staff had tied my hands down, making me a prisoner to my condition in my sterile accommodations. Now that it did not appear necessary to have it in place, the doctors wished to remove the tube as soon as possible to lessen my discomfort. The doctor had to first confirm my responsiveness.

"Neil, can you hear us? If you can, please give us some signal you understand," the doctor asked. "Squeeze my hand if you can understand me."

I remained still, with my eyes closed. After a couple more unsuccessful attempts to wake me, he resigned himself to the fact the tube would have to remain in place for the time being.

Mom was not as easily persuaded by my immobile posturing. She persisted and calmly but firmly said, "Neil, this is your mother speaking. Do you want that tube out of your throat? If you do, you have to wiggle your toes."

My toes began to move. To confirm this had not simply been a random occurrence, she continued, "If you want that tube out of your throat, squeeze my hand."

My hand immediately began to clench and unclench rapidly, and doctors liberated me from the tube.

With the wresting of control over my most basic bodily functions back from the machines, my healing began occurring at rapid rate, though numerous problems persisted. For those around me, it was an active process requiring significant amounts of assistance from unpaid observers.

My tongue began to return to its normal size and color, and my teeth began to slowly emerge from behind the receding swelling. To the surprise and great joy of my visitors, all of my teeth were still in my mouth. As my tongue continued to heal, Mom spent hours a day removing the dead flesh. Using star-shaped sponges dipped in mouthwash and affixed to a stick in the model of a Q-tip, she swabbed the rot out of my mouth to promote healing and to reduce the noxious odor that permeated the air around me. She went through bags of these each day. After she gently ran it around my mouth, the swab returned as a bloody mess, collecting the remnants of the damage from my tongue being bitten with such force during the wreck. In an attempt to minimize the permanence of my wounds, she also rubbed Vitamin E into the newly forming scars, which included some cuts from flying glass on my face and additional gashes on my feet, a product of being dragged out of the car and through the glass while wearing only flip-flops.

Even with all of the assistance provided to me, there were many remaining, seemingly insurmountable, hurdles. The trauma, followed by an intravenous diet, had ravaged my body and reduced my formerly 185 pound, relatively thin frame to a nausea-inducing 150 pounds of pasty skin stretched over protruding ribs. Nowhere on my body was an ounce of fat visible, and I took on the shape of a poorly stuffed scarecrow. Robbed of my natural insulation, my body was perpetually cold. My teeth chattered, especially at night, and I reflexively tried to find some way to stay warm, burrowed in the fetal position in the assorted blankets provided to me by the hospital staff.

Mom bought me a stuffed teddy bear she nicknamed 'Bama Bear, which I clung to throughout my remaining hospital stays and kept pressed up against me to retain whatever body heat I could. Amy delivered a Build-A-Bear named Chipper, after my favorite baseball player from childhood, and, dressed in an Atlanta Braves hat and a shirt reading "Someone in New Orleans Loves You," he joined in 'Bama Bear's quest to preserve my warmth. I was a grown man clinging to what would ordinarily be the vestiges of childhood in an attempt to survive.

Additional problems surfaced. I still remained incontinent, a less than thrilling proposition for the nurses in charge of changing my sheets. The nurses had other duties and patients on the floor and, since removing my soiled sheets was hardly their favorite activity, they frequently forsook it, leaving me to lie in my own waste. For Amy and Mom, this was entirely unacceptable. After observing how the nurses rolled the patients onto their sides in order to change the sheets, Mom and Amy took over yet another task: keeping my bedding clean.

The list of problems continued. I was too long for my bed, something which did not become a concern until I began to stabilize. At night, when I was curled up, this presented no issues; during the day, though, it led to less than thrilling moments for witnesses of both genders.

In order to situate my body in the bed, I continued to reflexively cross and uncross my legs, sometimes leaving them wide open. Ordinarily, this would not present any issues, but I was attired only in a hospital gown, and movements of this nature exposed all to views of my genitalia, often for prolonged periods of time. My visitors, mortified and uncomfortable upon witnessing my unthinking immodesty, quickly glanced away at the first signs of movement, but rarely in time to avoid the display. Their embarrassment was not shared by me, and they were forced to chuckle uncomfortably with their eyes staring at the ceiling as I lay comfortably with my legs splayed open. To limit my visitors' discomfort at their exposure to this salacious sight, the nurses rigged a sheet that hung across my knees and masked the offending area, thereby restricting their visiting experience to the R-rated macabre.

Despite the continued presence of these numerous issues, the fight began to return to me, and I slowly grew stronger. Two physical therapists began rehabilitation with me. Flanked by the therapists, one on either side to support me, I shuffled toward Mom and Amy with my unsupported head facing downward, wearily rolling side-to-side as I unevenly propelled myself in the direction of their cheering voices.

Since this was a busy trauma hospital staffed to keep people alive, not to assist them in their rehabilitation, the therapists had a very limited amount of time they could spend with me, generally about twenty minutes each day. During the walking sessions, Amy and Mom began paying attention to how the therapists supported me. Using the physical therapists' techniques they had observed during my prior walks, the two of them began supplementing my authorized walking sessions by walking me around the hospital two or three times during the day, stopping at the couches lining the wall at the end of the hall when I grew too tired. Each pass of the nurses' station found me pausing, as gregarious as the last time, and my eager waving, ear-to-ear grin and friendly, but high-pitched and nasal "hi" was always met with reciprocal warmth as they played along with the grinning boy who could not remember his last visit ten minutes prior. My left arm no longer functioned properly, but my balance became steadier, and if I was supported by one person, I could complete the walk that Mom insistently led me on with some degree of frequency.

Still, despite my physical progress, the problems with my mind were beginning to upset me even before I could retain memories. My identity was in my mind. My identity was my mind. I was the smart kid. I was.

During one of the walks with Mom, my brain, which was still only nominally functional, came to the realization that something was terribly wrong and began crowding out any remaining thoughts, leaving me to fixate on the newly perceived issue. I became despondent as I paused from dragging my semi-responsive legs around the ward and began hitting myself in the head. "I'm stupid!" I howled with the conviction of someone resigned to an inescapable fate.

"No, you aren't, you are smart," she tried to reassure me.

"I'm stupid! I'm stupid!" I slurred. "All my brains fell out."

Mom did her best to calm me down, responding, "No, you're smart," as soothingly as possible, knowing that I was echoing the fears of everyone around me. No one, least of all Mom, knew how much of my mind would come back, and she stood with me, trying to mask her own fears.

Concern continued to drive action by my invested observers, and everyone present participated in my rehabilitation. Kim, who had claimed her thankless role at the kitchen table in

Aiken, joined Mom and Amy in their volunteer job as daily rehabilitation coordinators. Kim's task was to return use to my left arm. She would lift my weak arm, and, with it aloft, encourage me to keep it raised. After I completed my valiant fight for whatever length of time I could and it returned to my side on the bed, she would request that I raise it on my own.

A few days after the accident, Kevin's girlfriend Rachel began to come to the hospital with my other visitors. She had a friend whose husband was involved in a car accident and had experienced a head trauma.

"They kept showing him pictures and reading him stories from magazines and books to get his brain started working again," Rachel told Mom and Amy. "He made a full recovery."

With the myth of a full recovery perpetuated, this became the goal of everyone around me, as they set out to fix my damaged brain. After my eyes had opened during the third day of my hospital stay, the information barrage never stopped. Amy printed out photos from our law school friend Joel Brewer's online photo gallery that documented graduation and other such events in which I had participated, and she constantly cycled through them, explaining to what event each photo pertained. The proof of who I was appeared before me, one still shot at a time.

The training continued and began to focus on my present ability to capture memories. The children's game of Memory emerged, and with Amy, Kim and Mom looking on and the smiling cartoon keys facing up, I tentatively pointed to one of their facedown brethren, expecting the friendly emancipators to greet me. I was so certain of my choice. When the card was flipped, I was entirely baffled by the fact that its twin remained hidden. My three trainers played along with me and provided thinly veiled hints to help my search, desperately hoping my accuracy would soon become statistically significant. But despite everyone's frustrations, there was no progress on this front—unbeknownst to my supportive participants, it wasn't time yet. None of them could imagine then how long these problems would continue to plague me.

{chapter 4}

Mom, Kim and Amy had transformed a trauma hospital room into my own personal rehabilitation hospital with hours of tireless work, but my continued presence there indicated that I had unfinished business at this site. Shortly after she first arrived at the hospital, Mom had consulted with numerous parties and chosen to postpone the plastic surgery necessary to repair the broken bones in my face until the surgeon regarded by many as the preeminent plastic surgeon in Alabama returned from his vacation. He was back in the office a week after Mom's initial attempt to contact him and, after speaking with her, he scheduled the surgery to repair my broken eye orbital and sinus cavity for ten o'clock one morning of the following week.

On the day the surgery was to occur, a series of individuals suffering from life-threatening injuries began to stream in, and their surgeries took precedence over mine. I had not eaten since midnight of the previous night, and it was soon eight o'clock that evening. The hospital staff spent the day warning Mom of his delays and then informed her it would be two in the morning before the surgery could take place. Concerned about both the doctor's fatigue and my need to eat, she requested they postpone until the following day, which they did, and I was at last allowed to eat.

The next morning, surgery commenced, and the doctor recreated a stable facial structure while imitating my prior appearance. With the addition of two mesh titanium plates, one inserted above my left eye and one below my right eye, he provided the bone a metal matrix around which it could grow. As a testament to his skill, the end result left a very small scar by my left eye where he entered to insert the corresponding plate, but no other evidence of a procedure. The past and the present promised to aesthetically intersect. I would look like I did before the wreck once the swelling subsided.

The world I occupied, though seemingly isolated from the events occurring all around it, was still at the mercy of what the walls and machines hid from view. Outside the hospital, Hurricane Ivan drew closer and was scheduled to make landfall and hit Mobile directly in the next two days. Mom assured Kim that, though her help had been invaluable, her continued presence in light of the coming storm was not advisable, and Kim found a flight out.

For Mom and Amy, departure was still not an option in their minds. After consulting with the staff, who assured them the hospital was the safest place in the area, since it had a back-up generator and water supply, they checked out of their hotel and moved into the facility. As midnight approached, Mom and Amy decided to get some sleep, knowing they would not likely find any opportunities for rest once the storm finally hit. Mom slept on the couch in my room and Amy slept on a pallet she had made.

When they woke, it was already morning. They cautiously parted the blinds, unsure of what they would see. The surrounding area looked normal. Surprised, they stopped a nurse who walked by.

"The hurricane veered at the last minute and hit the Florida Panhandle, and only the Northwest side of it struck Mobile."

They would learn throughout the morning that the storm still caused destruction, but it was not fully visible through the hospital window, and it was not as severe as forecasters had expected.

Since the primary outside distraction was of no further concern to the observers in my ward, their attention returned to me. The doctors re-evaluated my status, and Mom weighed in on the options offered. Despite the fact I remained in bad shape, my survival was no longer in doubt, and I needed to be moved to a rehabilitation hospital to continue my recovery.

The most promising facility, The Shepherd Center, which specialized in recovery from brain and spinal cord injuries, was located in Atlanta. When she learned that the wait to be admitted was six months, Mom moved to the next option and had me transferred to the Walton Rehabilitation Hospital in Augusta, Georgia, which also let her return to work at Aiken High School during the day.

But outside complications continued to interfere with everyone's plans. How I would get to Augusta was a mystery, since no ambulances remained available to transport me—they were all in use helping the local hurricane victims. Seeing no other way, Mom hired—at her own expense—an ambulance from Augusta, to drive down and bring me back to the rehabilitation hospital there.

My proposed residence was located in a city steeped in the traditions of my past. I had formerly visited Augusta as a celebratory retreat to mark a special occasion, be it birthday parties at the Chuck-E-Cheese, summer games played by the local Single-A baseball team, the Augusta Pirates, or shopping at the Augusta Mall for new school clothes. Three weeks after I entered the hospital in Mobile, an ambulance arrived to transport me to this city of my past. However, this journey did not allow for the unbridled excitement of an innocent child anxious to celebrate the passage of another mile marker. My speech remained barely coherent, and my frustrations, which had manifested themselves with regularity in the hospital, reappeared with unparalleled force during that ambulance ride.

Mom, having sent Amy back to New Orleans to check on everything there, was alone with staff trained to deal with the unwilling; she rode with me and one of the Emergency Medical Technicians in the back of the ambulance. The EMT was forced to restrain me before our departure, since I was angrily thrashing about, and he'd done so by tying me to a stretcher inside the vehicle. The restraints did not assuage my anger; I spent the entirety of the trip alternately trying to bite Mom and yelling obscenities at her, pausing only long enough to temporarily regain my strength so I could continue my fruitless struggle.

When we finally arrived in Augusta, I was exhausted from hours of fighting an unwinnable battle against my restraints, but neither my fatigue nor my physical limitations would inform my decisions. As they unstrapped me from the stretcher, I refused the wheelchair they had waiting for me, and with a nurse and Mom supporting me, I walked through the doors of Walton Rehabilitation Hospital.

{chapter 5}

Such a stumbling entrance into my new hospital indicated an unwillingness to accept my limitations, a trait that would serve me well throughout my rehabilitation. It also indicated how misaligned my perception of reality was. After the first day, when they helped me to my assigned room, I spent much of my unsupervised time trying to walk. Failure in this endeavor was inevitable, and my "walks" were frequent. Nurses returning to my room would frequently find me lying in a pile on the floor.

Concerned that I would fall and hit my head, they initially tied me to the bed before shifting me to a "veil bed," which prevented me from getting up and trying to walk around when I was unattended. After my initiation into the newest restraint device, my mourning began anew. The veil bed was an inescapable holding cell. It was a bed covered by netting that could only be unzipped from the outside, and it remained zipped at night.

"Please don't zip me in," I pleaded with Mom, night after night, as she readied herself to leave.

"I'm sorry, sweetie, I have to do this. It's just for the night. They will unzip you in the morning. Relax and go to sleep. I'll see you tomorrow."

My first memories were those of terror. Mom left and the darkness of a cage was the only thing I would know until morning. Fortunately, my fatigue was so powerful that what disquiet gripped me in the evenings lost out after less than an hour. But during that final hour, the paranoia raged. Something wasn't right.

"Someone at the hospital was trying to kill me," I whispered to Mom upon her return the following afternoon.

{the blocked path}

"No one is trying to kill you," she assured me, deeply concerned that my mind was failing me in new ways. In those moments, with the sunlight pouring in, still feeling relatively fresh after eleven hours of sleep the previous night, I could believe her. But as daylight began to fade, my anxiety increased and, upon Mom's departure the following night, the shadows of the netting across my still form reminded me of my powerlessness against the conniving hospital staff who stayed just out of my sight. This final waking hour became the most terrifying of my day during those veil bed stays. My mind, still too damaged to make sense of anything, had finally begun to record some events, and, unlike the frustration of my previous hospital stay, which belonged to my story tellers, this terror was mine to keep.

That I was now in a different city was of no import to me, especially in light of my nightly prison. With my new geographic location, though, changes began to occur. Amy was no longer a weekday fixture in my room, and Mom's presence did not simply reflect hospital visiting hours anymore. Mom was there every day directly after school, and, though Amy attended her law school classes Monday through Thursday afternoon in New Orleans, she arrived in Augusta Thursday night, or, if she was too tired to finish the drive, by Friday morning, guaranteeing I saw her by breakfast on Friday.

During the day, I found myself alone—left to think using the damaged device in my head, the biological equivalent of using a punch card computer in the Digital Age, and to heal, a passive process that they promised was occurring even while I felt nothing changing.

The hospital staff tried unsuccessfully to help me, but I grew tired of their efforts, which felt so pointless, and everyone around me felt my impotent wrath. On one occasion, a therapist arrived and requested synonyms for the word "short." I provided two words that worked, but she wanted more. Frustrated by her desire for more when I had nothing left, I improvised.

"Kurz," I finally responded.

The therapist looked at me strangely. Later, she would ask Mom about it, and Mom told her it was German.

"Do you think the he speaks German now because of the wreck?" the therapist then asked.

I was so sick of what I witnessed: the timid help offered and the inability of others to understand what was bothering me. How could these people not see the source of my frustrations? Weren't they trained to fix people like me? I wished to be anywhere but in that room, with its non-offensive color schemes and windows showing what I could not have, the shuffle of a passing nurse my only distraction from a life of barely living, meaning through existence alone. If only I was given another chance, I would never take any future opportunities for granted. I would not waste a second sleeping if I were set free from the regime that forced sleep by fiat. I would earn the future dividends I requested tomorrow. I would never take anything for granted. I would be better. The promises turned to pleas. I needed one more chance. No deal was struck, no answer was ever forthcoming. Instead, my words merely echoed around the empty halls of my head.

Luckily, though most days left me free to sit alone and promise God the assurances of penitence, Mom and Amy's less-frequent presence was supplemented by new faces. Brent, a friend from Aiken who had learned of my near-certain demise the day after the wreck occurred, was constantly visiting. He would arrive with his ever-present enthusiasm and energy to entertain me in whatever manner he could determine that day. My friend Cory, another former Aiken compatriot, travelled in from Columbia on occasion to see me, too.

Karen, curious as to why I had not made my promised journey to Baltimore, left numerous messages on my cell phone, a device lost to the hills surrounding I-65. After not receiving a response to her previous inquiries, she began to investigate more thoroughly. When she was finally able to reach my mother, who was now back at her house in Aiken, she learned the news and came down to see me one weekend. In Augusta, Karen spent parts of the day observing one of my painfully limited rehabilitation sessions and played board games with me, including Monopoly, where she and Amy threw themselves into the task of losing with the gusto generally reserved for the homes of parents with young children.

My friend Shawn Carlson even made the trip from Hawaii to join my growing group of visitors, watching football one Saturday and visiting with me during his time back in the Continental United States. We sat watching UVA football one Saturday, and he made small talk with me.

"You doing okay today?" he asked.

"I am so tired," I answered, pausing ever so slightly before offering my logical conclusion as to why I was so fatigued. "I've been Chinese antiquing all day, and I am exhausted."

{chapter 6}

And so, as my face returned to its normal size and I began to resemble who I had once been, friends from my more distant past were all around me. I was able to speak, and my brain functions were coming back online, though still painfully slowly at times. A very limited version of my self-awareness began to appear.

One of my hang-ups had always been using public restrooms to defecate. As my bowel control finally returned, I learned that someone was required to be in the restroom with me to ensure I did not fall over and hit my head while I sat on the toilet, a far more invasive proposition than having someone in the stall next to me.

I held out, hoping the required monitoring rule would be rescinded, but my physical progress was insufficient to allow for this. Thus, after considering my options, I relented and proceeded into the bathroom with my chaperone.

I sat on the commode and tried to ignore the person who stood in the corner. My abdomen ached with a pain reminiscent of my experience during the long car rides returning from visiting my grandparents in Louisville. But the relief at the end of the trip was no longer available to me. The presence of another in the bathroom was something I just could not blindly ignore; so after sitting on the toilet for a few minutes without making any further efforts for the observing staff member, who was attempting to blend in with the surrounding tile, I flushed and departed. My behavior alarmed the nurses, who worried that there was a physiological reason for my constipation.

During Karen's visit, the nurse pulled Amy aside. "We have been pumping your boyfriend full of laxatives, and we can't get him to poop. Can you see what you can do about it?"

"Of course he won't. He hates public restrooms." She and Karen then wandered through the hospital until they came upon a private restroom in a seldom-used part of the hospital.

The two of them put me into a wheelchair and wheeled me down to their latest discovery.

"Is this restroom big enough?" Amy asked.

"Yes," I said quickly, before entering and closing the door.

The two of them stood guard, trying to muffle their laughter, as days of laxatives finally bore results, and my body reacted with such fervor that the repercussions were fully audible to the two women standing outside.

Mom remedied my problem in the subsequent days by asking on occasion that she be allowed to sign me out for a few hours, and the hospital staff always approved her request to do so. We arrived home, where I rushed into the house and headed straight to the bathroom. With her outside the closed door to monitor me, I was able to relieve myself in peace.

My daytime mobility brought with it the privilege of once again bathing myself. Still, as was becoming obvious to everyone including me, privacy was not an option when I was still so fragile, and the sources of my embarrassment remained the domain of the staff in charge of protecting me.

I was not trusted to shower on my own, despite the fact my bathing could take place from the seated convenience of a broad mesh chair which folded out from the wall. With my faculties returning, I found this nearly as humiliating as my bathroom monitoring. On one occasion, accompanied by a female nurse, I was seated in the mesh chair attached to the wall and letting the water run off me while I applied soap liberally across my emaciated form, when I noticed I was being assisted. Though this sounds like a fantasy, I did not find it remotely alluring and was instead shocked by her intrusion.

She calmly explained I was missing spots, an assertion that, while undoubtedly true, was entirely irrelevant to me at that moment. After my horrified reaction, she resumed observing to ensure I did not fall off the seat, but did not intervene any further.

Not all of my observers were of the professional variety. Uncertain tomorrows had made me popular, and the hospital was kind enough to accommodate my weekend flood of visitors. In the main common room, there were televisions that could be tuned in to college football and, one Saturday, my guests were treated to the viewing of a UVA football game. Unfortunately, despite the healing that had taken place already, I was still not fully coherent.

During my walks around the hospital with Mom, I had begun trying to engage various workers—responsible for washing windows and the like—in conversation about a variety of football teams that I believed I was coaching. Accustomed to residents who were not fully functional, they readily ignored me while Mom encouraged me to leave the men alone and to keep walking.

During this particular Saturday game viewing, I knew myself to be coaching UVA. My present borrowed from my past, but only so far as it was convenient. Using terminology acquired from years of PlayStation NCAA and Madden football games, I barked orders at the television that, to my chagrin, were never followed and, I later learned, were complete nonsense.

"This is part of the healing process and is not particularly worrying. We will watch it to make sure it doesn't get worse," a doctor explained to Mom when she raised her concerns. As he predicted, the hallucinations continued but did not worsen.

Though Mom felt reassured by the doctor's explanation, I had also stopped eating, which was a far more pressing concern.

My jaw was aching, and since dull pain was part of my daily routine anyway, I did not deem this issue to be noteworthy. When the jaw pain became sharp and persistent, I finally chose to notify the staff. They presented me with the 1-10 pain scale. I wisely avoided the hyperbolic twenty.

"Seven."

The flurry of activity began. No one chose seven. The nurses frenetically responded to a number that indicated both pain and an acceptance of the idea that the pain could be worse than it was at that moment. Since no cause could be found, the prescribed treatment of painkillers simply tackled the symptom.

The new daily numbness blurred the lines between dreams and reality. I had to pinch myself while awake to confirm what I was seeing was real, though even with such confirmation, I never felt like I was awake.

The issues with my jaw finally culminated in an event that demanded a solution. One day I yawned, but it would not depart with the peacefulness with which it arrived. Its continued presence implied permanence, and I began to struggle to snap my jaw shut as I sat in my bed with my mouth agape. I clenched harder, but to no avail. Nurses were summoned. The fear in my eyes reflected the silent scream that was pasted on my face. Their initial instructions proved unhelpful, and they began to inspect me more closely. As my mouth remained open, my spit turned to paste.

"Just relax, Sweetie," one of the nurses gently encouraged.

Relaxation was a simple concept, but it proved difficult for me to implement when my mouth was stuck open. After a few minutes, an enterprising nurse placed both index fingers in my mouth parallel to my jaw line and pushed back while lifting up. My jaw slipped back into place and my mouth finally closed. This relief proved necessary time and again, as the contagion of even a stifled yawn would send me back to this horrendous state. My visitors were warned not to yawn around me, which guaranteed they would do precisely that. Due to the repetitive nature of this issue, the nurses taught Mom how to reset my jaw in a manner that would avoid me biting her fingers.

These incidents clearly indicated that something was wrong with yet another part of my face. I was sent to the maxillofacial surgeon Dr. Howell, who had removed my wisdom teeth after my first year of college. He was a relatively young doctor who chatted amicably at me as he explored my mouth. He took an x-ray of my teeth, and the image he inspected confirmed that two teeth, an incisor and back molar on the right side, were dead, due to damaged roots, so he used a localized anesthetic and removed them. The revelations continued when, after further inspection of the x-ray, he came to the startling realization that my right jaw line had two additional fractures.

This meant that a section of my jaw was not firmly attached to the surrounding bone, and this floating bone fragment was slipping out and striking a nerve along my jaw line, triggering my jaw to clench. In addition to this, the jaw orbital, which served as the hinge on the right side of my face, was chipped, leaving its circular joint incomplete and allowing it to pop out of socket. The combination of these two injuries and certain facial movements, such as yawning, resulted in my jaw clenching with such force that it freed itself from the chipped orbital and came to a rest below its former joint, preventing the hinge from once again closing.

Though this injury had been noted by medical staff in Alabama, with the plethora of other issues present and the intense facial swelling it had been forgotten. Now, even while my face healed, my improving outward appearance simply masked the unpleasantness that lay below the surface. The medical explanation offered by Dr. Howell with the aid of his x-ray map was certainly beyond me and of little help to Mom.

We both understood the conclusion it led to, though— more surgery was necessary to correct this problem, and it was scheduled at a different hospital. The surgery, he explained to me, would include placing a plate along my right jaw line to stabilize the jaw and let it heal back together and then drilling a screw through the right jaw orbital to ensure that it would never dislocate again.

My undergoing yet another surgery was not what anyone was hoping for, but I lived in constant fear of yawning and this problem would not correct itself. My reluctance to eat was also explained by the breaks, since chewing on a broken jaw was an unpleasant experience, even for someone accustomed to pain. Thus, this problem, too, seemed likely to disappear after the surgery and subsequent period of healing.

The procedure was scheduled at a hospital associated with the Medical College of Georgia, and it took place at the arranged time. After surgery, they moved me to a recovery room and armed me with the most potent weapon against pain I have ever experienced, a morphine drip. I had to press a button to have my IV release additional morphine, and, should my requests exceed the medically allowed dosage, it would beep at me and refuse to dispense any more until the appropriate time had passed, to prevent me from overdosing. It was perfect—medically controlled escapism. With continued pressing of the button, I wouldn't know where I was, but I wouldn't care.

The day after the surgery, I vacillated between indescribable euphoria and a hell where I experienced pain unequaled by anything I'd ever felt. The halls echoed with the beep of my defiant drug dealer; I pressed the button without regard to its willingness to dispense additional medication, as if my thumb was a rogue agent no longer under my command. The feeling that morphine delivered was the closest thing to pure pleasure I have ever experienced, and I was floating, unaware of anything else, basking in its glow. The harsh world that awaited me upon my departure ensured that there would not be any failure on my part to request further prescription refills.

By the next morning, I was returned to Walton Hospital. A week later, after my follow-up visit with Dr. Howell when he pronounced my surgery a success, I scheduled an appointment with the same orthodontist who had shepherded my teeth into line during my teen years to now install braces that would rubber band my mouth shut and allow my jaw to fully heal.

Once again, my orthodontist equipped me with the aesthetically captivating sight of a mouth full of metal, but this time my mouth was additionally sealed shut with a series of rubber bands attached to my upper and lower jaws. I returned to the hospital having completed my transformation into a gangly teenager, my mouth now matching my spindly physique.

I had participated in the hospital's inpatient rehabilitation classes from the moment I arrived in Augusta, and the physical therapists noted my marked improvement as time passed. I practiced walking up two free standing stairs and engaged in light exercise, moving from station to station in the hospital's small gym while under the watchful eye of resident physical therapists. With the last of my surgeries behind me, I continued to show improvement, and the doctors began discussing discharging me to an outpatient treatment facility.

Amy was in town when I learned the good news that, after two months of hospital beds, I would finally be allowed to sleep away from the tired eyes of night shift nurses and the vigilant monitoring of cold machines. As we walked around outside the hospital in advance of my final day, I moved purposefully along the abandoned railroad tracks that ran behind the hospital while Amy walked beside me to help steady me if I wobbled. Eventually, we arrived at the hospital's children's playground. I climbed to the top of the slide and sat down to survey the surrounding area.

Sitting there in the sun on that clear fall day, my future finally felt promising again. I thought I was so close to reclaiming it all, something Mom had stubbornly predicted would occur, even when doctors were initially disinclined to believe her. At the time of my arrival at Walton, my stay was to be six weeks. I was being discharged in three. I was once again at the head of my class.

There was reason to hope, better yet, to know that I would be fine. This was going to require one last push, one final bit of hard work, and then I thought I could simply resume my life, armed with a story that would awe listeners at cocktail parties. I thought it would all be over soon. In retrospect, that was a belief cloaked in naivety. Far too many of my memories and abilities had disappeared for my recovery to be this easy.

{chapter 7}

The following week, I was discharged from the hospital and began spending my days at the out-patient rehabilitation facility. This facility specialized in reintegrating injured individuals back into the community. The age of the participants varied greatly, though I was one of the youngest. One of my former roommates from Walton Rehabilitation Hospital also participated in out-patient rehabilitation there. He was approximately twenty when his car had been t-boned by an eighteen-wheeler, and he was a couple of weeks ahead of me in his rehabilitation. He and I would spend many of our afternoons after lunch shooting baskets on the hoop behind the center or throwing the football. It was during those times, when our morning activities were complete and the afternoon chores had not yet begun, that we both got to be carefree kids for a few minutes of the day, irrespective of our relative athleticism—no one from the outside world was present to mock us or to compare his fluid ease with my ever-present clumsiness.

The degree of freedom this facility afforded me was incredible, since I was no longer confined to a hospital bed, though the rehabilitation center still maintained a structured rotation of activities conducted by various staff members. We went with them to the grocery store and bought the items necessary to make whatever recipe we had chosen to cook for lunch. When the group to which I was assigned was responsible for making the day's meal, I worked with my team to prepare the balanced meal we designed, though it was a meal I still could not eat because of my jaw.

Each of the rehabilitation clients met with a speech pathologist on an individual basis to adjust our pronunciation and focus on our enunciation. Throughout the day, we engaged in a variety of other activities as well, including a trip to a local pumpkin patch where we selected pumpkins, and then, under the watchful eye of staff members, carved our simple jack-o-lanterns. A couple of times a week, we were given access to a small nearby gym, which included weight machines and a treadmill.

At night, I returned to the house in which I grew up. I had not permanently lived at home since I was eighteen years old, and I grew late in high school. I had outgrown my bed by the time I left for college, but the immediacy of my departure meant there was no need to purchase a new one. Returning to my old home meant that I was returning to a twin bunk bed that did not provide room enough for me to sit up fully while I was on the bottom bunk and was approximately six inches shorter than I was. Mom quickly saw the need to remedy this problem. We visited Macy's during their mattress sale the following weekend, and, after I lay on the various available mattresses to determine which one was best suited for me, I chose (and she purchased) a queen-sized extended Sealy bed that would accommodate my height and helped lessen some of the lower back pain I'd begun experiencing during my extended hospital stays.

As my accommodations were now entirely suitable for me, the logistics of my stay became the predominant concern. The scheduling issues were not remotely vexing to me, but Mom's adjustment was significant, since I still had so many problems requiring attention. She was still alarmed by my previous weight loss, since I had only managed to regain ten pounds in the interim, and my weight rested at an only slightly more respectable 160 pounds, still far underweight for someone my height. Mom decided she had to figure out ways to put weight back on me, in spite of my inability to eat solid food because of my broken jaw.

{the detours}

My morning routine began to take shape. Mom woke early and prepared shakes by throwing whole milk, whipped cream, ice cream, strawberries, peaches, bananas, Ensure, and, occasionally, pieces of cheesecake, into the blender, and, after a minute of noisy comingling, when it was devoid of sizable chunks, she would pour it into a glass and demand that I consume it in its entirety before I departed for my day. After finishing my shake, I would gently brush my teeth. Then, for the next ten minutes, she would help me put the rubber bands in place while I squirmed around, annoyed and agitated by the whole process, which was a further reminder of my helplessness. After this process was complete, she then packed me off for rehab with a variety of high calorie protein and other meal replacement shakes, and one of our neighbors would take me to Augusta, while Mom hurriedly tried to finish preparing for her school day. After Mom finished school, she would arrive to pick me up, frequently bearing a Frusion yogurt shake or other such drink meal supplement that I would consume through a straw while she asked me about my day.

Initially, the conversations on our ride home were brief. Memories were still disappearing too quickly to allow for transmittal to others. I would distill my eight-hour day into one sentence that described one activity.

"Think back," she would instruct. "What else did you do today? Did you go to the gym? Did your group cook? Did you go to the store?"

I had told her everything, I would insist, my anger and frustration bubbling to the surface, before she quickly changed the subject to calm me down.

Gradually, my recollection of the day's events began to include more and more information as my short-term memory began to return. Even in a day with many activities rigidly scheduled, there was a lot of free time. I spent some of it on the Internet, emailing friends and sometimes other people with whom I hadn't communicated in years. I also spent much of the day talking to the others who were rehabbing there, learning about what I had never had to wrestle with on a daily basis before—loss.

It became clear as the details emerged from hiding that my time in rehab was more than just a period of escape from other people's judgment while I tried to regain my faculties. My days there were forcing me to actively observe the lives of people who were less fortunate than anyone I had known before; but I was not a voyeur peering in through the window. I bore the hospital discharge paperwork that showed I belonged. The staff invited me in, and my fellow residents knew me as one of them. Everyone, including me, was clearly still injured, and we were at different points on our road to recovery.

The stories they told were incredible, unlike anything I had ever heard. As time went on, more and more made the return trip home with me and Mom, though many details of my daily interaction with them still did not survive. My new universe was a place where everyone had a story, and my eyes were briefly opened to the pain of others. Their stories would stick, even though other details and concepts would not.

A nice woman in her late twenties or early thirties, who was a mother of two, told me that when she was parachuting three years before, her parachute had opened late. It had cushioned her landing enough for her to survive, but the fall had broken numerous bones and left her with debilitating injuries. She was fighting to be able to return home to her family, which she was successful in doing before I completed my time there.

Another woman had been riding in her boyfriend's truck when, in an act of senseless violence, a group of teens had dropped a cinder block over the overpass and in of the truck. The block went through the windshie through her face. Her boyfriend sped on to the r pulled into the first gas station there, panicking ar them to call 911, but they had already done so, as she had part of her brain on the front of her shirt and her face wore the sickening trauma of flesh and bone impacting an immovable object at high speed. They performed surgery to save her and cosmetic surgery to repair her face, but still, despite the fact that she was twenty-six when I met her, she spoke and acted like she was fifteen, with an inappropriate air of sexuality that she would sporadically exude. From what I could tell, she would remain the emotional equivalent of a teenager for the rest of her life. She was once featured on Montel Williams, understandably a source of great pride for her.

A guy a year or two my senior was another member of my class with whom I spoke frequently. He had previously worked in construction, and since he showed no fear of heights, he was usually assigned tasks on the upper stories of the buildings in the area that his employer was constructing. The safety belt that secured him slowed him down, and neither he nor his supervisors saw the need for him to wear it at all times. One day, while working on a building, he slipped and fell. The fall broke his spine. He was then, and would forever remain, confined to a wheelchair, though he still spoke of life in the carefree manner reflective of a twenty-year-old frat kid. About once every two weeks, when we made our trip to a nearby pool hall in the dreaded bus that humiliatingly announced us as "special," he would emerge from the vehicle by way of the automated back platform and patiently keep our team competitive, despite virtually no help from me.

Another man there in his early forties was formerly part of a motorcycle gang and had the ink and hair to prove it. He went over the handlebars of his bike one day, and, not equipped with a helmet, did irreparable damage both to his body and his brain. He had lost over 100 pounds from his days in the bike gang, and when his tough guy persona surfaced, which it did ery once in a while, it was painful to witness, as his physical stature no longer lent any intimidating power, and his broken speech did not instill fear.

A recent retiree from St. Simons Island was another addition to our group. He had fallen from a ladder while cleaning his gutters and hit his head. Every day, anyone within earshot would learn of how perfect St. Simons Island was and how he longed to return with his wife to his house there. I found it callous that he bemoaned the loss of some of his retirement years, when so many of the people by whom we were surrounded would never have the opportunity to live independently without significant financial and social support. Still, I could understand his frustration with the loss of the opportunities he had worked his entire life to earn, and, despite my early reluctance to accept the merits of his complaints, I began to appreciate where he was coming from, even while I rapidly tired of hearing about St. Simons Island.

Of all of the stories I shared with Mom on my return trek home, the only individual who did not elicit sympathy from me during my telling was a permanent resident who had the most severe injuries. He walked with the assistance of a walker, which he used to unevenly propel himself about the facility, and though he retained the ability to be friendly, he rarely implemented it. He was heavy-set, but more husky than fat, though the staff was forever monitoring his eating habits.

I do not know what happened to him. He joined us for rehabilitation during the day, but unlike most of us, he also lived at the facility, and his family sporadically visited. He was prone to violent outbursts, and the rumor that circulated among the other residents was that his family, equipped with the financial means and unsure of how to handle him, sent him there to keep him from harming anyone else. As he was a prominent source of funds, the staff tried to placate him as best as they could; their rebukes rarely carried more threatening language than the loss of dessert privileges. He called female residents fat and ugly, and he staggered head-on into confrontations, raising his voice in the most threatening manner possible toward anyone who chose to oppose him.

I soon became aware of his status as the tyrannical bully, and began to occasionally challenge him when I felt he had crossed lines. I generally kept quiet, but in those select moments, I denied him the affirmation his implicit authority had previously garnered him. If I was part of the group cooking and he demanded free access to the occupied kitchen, I informed him this was not an option. Though I remained convinced that my actions were for the benefit of others, these tragi-comic encounters empowered me to believe my presence there was in some way important.

Upon hearing these stories, Mom asked that I let the staff handle the situation and not become confrontational with a seriously handicapped individual, regardless of what he'd done, recognizing my ability to mete out social justice was limited, and my concept of the term "justice" was likely skewed. For the most part, I followed her directive and avoided these situations whenever possible.

As is the case with most chaperoned groups, we often had periods of time when our silence was requested, when I could not pass the time listening to other people's stories, and the staff directed us to quietly play board games or read. I had generally found reading enjoyable since childhood, so I perused what material was available to me. My first encounter with the printed word demonstrated yet another problem: the words on the page swam together and were rendered completely illegible. I alerted some of the social workers at the facility to my problem, and they suggested I use a ruler to set off the line I was trying to read. Upon implementing their suggestion, the words came into focus. My brain had forgotten how to compile the separate images fed from each of my eyes, and the ruler would retrain them by the end of my stay.

{the blocked path}

My next discovery was in the field of head injuries. A manual on the shelves of the facility discussed the medical implications of brain injury, and I began to review it, hoping to glean some helpful information. I learned that sometimes these injuries caused changes in personal temperament and some people found that they would become angry or frustrated more easily. The revelation about injury symptoms seemed to reflect what I had noticed about myself and my fellow participants during my time in rehabilitation.

What I read next elicited such a reaction from me. A couple of days before, one of the female social workers, who was an attractive, tall, blonde woman about two years older than me, was interviewing me to determine how I was doing.

"Have you noticed any changes since your wreck?" she asked.

"Yes," I had said in hushed tones, clearly embarrassed by the revelation that was to follow. "I am incredibly horny all of the time."

The look on her face was one of complete horror. "That is not appropriate! Please do not say things like that."

Shame had followed immediately, some portion of it offered as an apology and the rest retained to prevent any other such future indiscretions. She had offered neither sympathy nor understanding when I had provided my honest answer, but I had blamed myself for the misstep. Yet there, on the page open before me listing the side effects of a brain injury was an "increased sex drive." I had been chastised for describing a symptom of my condition. Of course, another symptom was the injured individual acting in a socially inappropriate manner, which I presume was the behavior she was attempting to remedy, but my righteous indignation remained for far too long.

I found myself living in this new world, with its unusual occupants and crazy problems, and was anxious to get out, but most days I was quietly resigned to the fact that this was all I was allowed to have. I tried to look forward to the trips to Wal-mart or my liquid lunches. I learned to smile at boredom and depression, and the arch on my jump shot did improve through mindless repetition during my recess reprieve, where I tried to dream my childhood dreams of NBA stardom as the ball fell through the net. But reality would not let this happen. Any daydreams were interrupted by my frequent dizziness or a call to return inside.

And so the dull daily routine continued, until one afternoon, there was a deviation from the norm. Mom arrived early, bearing a large cake. She was smiling, the same smile she wore to both of my graduations, and after I was notified of her approach by one of the staff, I walked out to meet her.

"Congratulations, Counselor," she said, her voice welling with pride. She walked inside with me, her hands full before depositing the cake on a nearby table, and showed me the letter from the Georgia Board of Bar Examiners. Neil Christopher Ligon had passed the bar and, after being sworn in, would be a licensed attorney in Georgia. My fellow residents gathered around for cake and looked at me, visibly impressed.

"You are a lawyer now?" someone asked.

"What kind of lawyer are you going to be?" another questioned.

I was relieved, since I had proclaimed to all that I had failed, both immediately following the exam and during the weeks before I was notified of the result. How would I study for a test of such magnitude without a working short-term memory? But now, after months of embarrassing incidents and pathetic displays, when I felt shame every time I stumbled into a room, no matter the location, I finally had something that announced my significance to all. This was how it was supposed to happen. The swagger returned, and I explained to everyone, through my rubber-banded teeth, that I was going to be a transactional real estate attorney.

{the blocked path}

The blank stares that greeted my response mirrored my own ignorance as to what this actually meant. The precise details were unimportant. I was going to be rich and successful. That was what kind of lawyer I was going to be. I removed my rubber bands and gingerly forced the cake down. It was only a matter of time before I returned to my journey and became who I was supposed to be.

Spurred on by my bar passage, I knew that I had only a few remaining hurdles before I returned to my life in Atlanta. I went into overdrive, and I focused all aspects of my life on using every waking hour to accelerate my recovery. The movies I watched on the weekends involved people without their memory struggling against unknown antagonists. Unarmed with a villain of my own, I channeled their anger into my own fight.

No one had left me to die on the side of the road; my decisions, rain and bad luck had put me there. But the wounded warrior I watched in Man on Fire—his vengeance spoke to me as I churned through another set of twenty pushups or 100 crunches, much as Jason Bourne's efforts would spur me on later that day. Disjointed memories were speed bumps, fractured images could all be pieced together through effort, and I would emerge victorious. After only one unsettling viewing, Memento was excluded.

My new taste in music allowed only for death metal and hardcore rap, and their resonating bass and defiant lyrics spit vengeance into my ears as I joined Mom in her trips to her gym in the evenings, where I threw myself into my workouts, pushing myself until I could feel every muscle of the targeted group burn from fatigue. The contrast between my suburban recovery and my imagined universe of danger and revenge did not affect my resolve, momentarily borrowed from others' worlds.

{the detours}

During my weekdays in rehab, my gym time remained a focused effort, whether straining with a lat pulldown bar anchored to plates that equaled my weight or matching the treadmill's rapid pace, my feet pounding its unforgiving thin rubber track as the digital distance on the screen in front of me ticked upward.

I religiously worked on the balance board, a plastic board with only a medium-sized rubber ball in its center to support it, in an attempt to regain my balance. While standing on the board, any significant wobbling, if it were not rapidly adjusted for, resulted in the board tipping and the standing party having to step off onto the floor to steady himself. I was determined that I would soon be able to stand on it unmoved by instability. My old hospital roommate had mastered this, and I vowed to someday better him in this task.

My workouts began to show results, but not always in the manner I expected. With the loss of weight, I remained too thin, but my work resulted in my regaining some of the muscle definition from my younger years. Unfortunately, my body was not entirely up for the effort, and the side effects of my final push included shin splints, leaving me to rub ice over the front of my legs after my return from the gym and limiting my running significantly until they could heal further.

With this setback, I focused on other efforts. One weekend I went on driving lessons with Mom's boyfriend at the time. He valiantly suffered through my struggles to maintain the car's location within the lane and calmly cautioned me about using my mirrors and the like. Upon our return, he proclaimed me once again fit to drive, and I was enrolled in a driving class, which made his assessment official after a few sessions.

I began playing tennis once a week in the evenings with a couple of men who were wheelchair-bound. My advantage was obvious: I was the only one able to walk. But my balance frequently betrayed me, I could not track the ball while it was in flight unless I was stationary, and my hand-eye coordination remained woefully inadequate, rendering me the weakest of the players. I grew frustrated knowing I had once been very good. Upon returning home to my room, adorned with tennis plaques celebrating tournament wins and notable finishes, I looked around at all the success before settling down on the edge of my bed. There, right in front of me, a tennis ball scarred with red ink from my old Wilson sponsorship stencil rested in a three-pronged holder whose base read "1996 AAAA State Champions." I wanted so badly to still be the guy on that court in Columbia, blasting serve after serve while my partner put away our opponents' weak returns, my partner and I trying so hard to suppress the smiles that we could feel rising, knowing that we were unstoppable and that we would soon be declared the best team in the state.

All the reminders of my past fed my revulsion about who I had become. I had once been almost impressive for a small-town South Carolina kid, but every day something showed me I wasn't him anymore. The evening's melancholy eventually faded, and I returned to the courts the next week, and my fellow drill participants again did not take exception to my inclusion in our coached drills or my outbursts born of frustration. My Wednesday nights were henceforth reserved for playing tennis under the lights on nearby courts.

As my workouts began to diversify, I resumed attempts to remedy my intellectual shortcomings as well. Armed with the ruler, I picked up a Clive Cussler book, as I had always enjoyed his stories, and consumed lighter fare of the sort for a period of time. Not finding much else that interested me, I mentioned to Mom and Amy that I was looking for things to read, and soon they were both offering me books that they thought would be suitable. One of Amy's selections, David Sedaris' Me Talk Pretty One Day, was particularly timely, as I was working with my speech pathologist in earnest to correct my lazy speech and reading of Sedaris's unfixable lisp was both funny and familiar.

I was, at that very moment, experiencing a parallel frustration. My speech pathologist was growing impatient with me, as I was showing no progress in my ability to properly articulate the letter "r." One afternoon, during our meeting, she looked at me more closely.

"Do you think your problems pronouncing these words have anything to do with those rubber bands and braces?" she asked. I, too, had previously been at a loss for the reasons behind my struggles. This theory had never occurred to me, but it made perfect sense.

I nodded my head vigorously, and punctuated the motion with a relieved, "Yes."

After that conclusion was reached, future speech therapy sessions were terminated, as the physiological culprit could not be eliminated for another couple of weeks and trying to remedy the unfixable was not a suitable use of either of our times.

But even with my mouth full of metal, the greatest obstacle to my communication efforts remained my mind. Long pauses marred my speech as I searched in vain for the word that perfectly captured the idea to which my latest sentence was committed. Ever so slight upper body sways hoped to purge from my mouth the word trapped in my head, though it remained lodged with the tenacity of an embedded tick.

"Just choose another word, Neil," Mom would gently implore me, but such surrender seemed premature when I knew the force of that mystical word would soon be mine. The reinforcements never arrived, and I would choose a weaker word and resume my meandering story, regretting my choice by the time the next syllable left my lips. As my time in rehab began to draw to a close, the pauses grew less frequent and no longer threatened to muddle the meaning of the sentences.

{the blocked path}

The hesitancy became only a minor inconvenience, which I thought, like the braces, would eventually disappear.

That December, I traveled to Atlanta for my swearing in ceremony at the Georgia Supreme Court, the final step in making me a lawyer. As I stood with my palm raised and repeated the oath to the Court with my legal counterparts, I remembered every word, and dutifully repeated it in unison with the surrounding new lawyers. I was officially a licensed attorney.

After the ceremony, still armed with braces and missing a visible tooth, I visited with one of the guys who interned with me two summers previously and the partner for whom I would be working, Eric Hale.

"Glad to hear you're ok. You had us worried there! We're really looking forward to you starting with us in January," Eric boomed. "We're going to have you start part time, and, after you get adjusted, we'll move you to full time."

He continued on, detailing the happenings at the law firm I still had yet to join. My friend Todd was being sent abroad to work in the firm's new Paris office despite not speaking a word of French. The firm's personnel had turned over, as firm employees customarily did. The real estate market in Atlanta was thriving, and the group was incredibly busy. During my absence, they'd hired four new associates, two of the more senior level and two junior associates, one of whom was only a year ahead of me in school and had worked at Eric's former firm. As I listened to him summarize the happenings at the firm, I thought Eric was delivering the blueprint for my life. My job was simply to build what was being shown to me.

I returned home to Aiken, having tasted what awaited me and itching to return to Atlanta. The speed with which time flew by was dizzying. My braces came off before Christmas, so my smile no longer advertised my previous trauma, outside my missing tooth, a problem my dentist scheduled to remedy in January with a bridge. The final weeks in Aiken were a formality, and Mom gathered my remaining belongings in preparation for my departure after Christmas. We ate our traditional Christmas meal with the Stone family, and my Christmas presents, already numerous, included a promised shopping spree at Mom's expense once we got to Atlanta, to buy me clothes for my important job.

On December 28, we left for Atlanta, and I moved my remaining stuff into my awaiting apartment, the same apartment I had lived in the summer I took the bar and for which Mom had dutifully been paying the rent, in spite of its vacancy. As Eric had explained to me during my swearing-in ceremony, I was to begin my job part time, with the intention that I become full time after a short trial period. Mom and I visited Joseph A. Banks, and she purchased assorted shirts and slacks that I chose for work and had my other pants taken in to accommodate my weight loss. I returned to my apartment, new shirts in hand and tickets for the pants being altered.

I visited the leasing office and picked up the packages that had been delivered in my absence. Amy had enrolled me in a beer of the month club for my twenty-fifth birthday, and an assortment of micro-brews awaited me. I placed them in my cupboard for storage, since I was not to drink alcohol yet because of the brain injury. We reviewed the bus and the train routes, since my totaled Explorer was now property of the insurer, and she printed out the route to ensure I would remember it. We found a dry cleaning store that I could walk to. She located the appropriate bus stop up the street on Peachtree Road for me.

Mom continued to tinker around the apartment as the time for her to leave drew closer, straightening any clutter and repeating the messages that she always shared with me prior to every one of her departures since her trips back to Aiken from Charlottesville, Virginia, seven and a half years ago.

"You will do great things. Stay organized. Get your rest. Don't forget to eat, and please eat salads, too. I love you, and I am so proud of you."

But her trepidation reflected a new reality, one where her absence would initially only be temporary.

"I will be back in two weekends. You have my number. If you need anything, call me. I do not care what time it is, call me."

Scared but excited, I was prepared to resume my life. I watched her leave and spent my first night in four months as an independent person with my stomach in knots, unsure of what to expect next, but knowing it would be better than what I had seen over the last four months. I had worked my way back, and though it had been a long and trying detour, I thought the hard part was complete. Rehab provided me with the necessary systems to conquer the obstacles. If I could sort out one or two little things, I thought I would get to start again where I had left off the previous summer. Reality was about barge in, and it would soon disavow me of this simple-minded belief.

*it
looked
familiar*

{chapter 8}

The first days of work were less about work and more an introduction to an entirely new world, the world I had dreamed of since my third year in law school. I signed the forms presented to me by human resources and stopped by the nearby offices, including the managing partner's office, to say hello. I swung by the offices on other floors, chatting briefly with the people whom I had known as a summer intern, and then made rounds to meet the people with whom I would be working. Of the individuals in the Real Estate group whom I knew from my summer internship, there were only three remaining—Eric, a senior associate named Jay, and Susan, a paralegal who had worked with Eric for twenty years. I was ushered around our portion of the twenty-third floor of the building to say my hellos.

After the meet and greet, I re-entered the office that they indicated would be mine. It was amazing. For someone who had only held summer jobs, the fact I had an office that would soon have a nameplate in front of it, marking it as mine, made me feel like an adult. The back wall was entirely glass, and as I sat in my chair and rotated around to face it, I looked out from twenty-three stories up onto the city of Atlanta. There was no denying that I had arrived; I needed only to turn around at my desk for proof of my accomplishments.

My hours were restricted to ten to three, but during my somewhat abbreviated day, I could witness work distribution and soon became acquainted with office politics. Each partner had a senior level associate who worked primarily for him, and there were a number of more inexperienced attorneys who were used by whoever needed them, though the more senior associates grew accustomed to working with particular younger associates, and, if their work product was strong, called upon them with greater frequency. The partner's primary responsibility was to elicit business from his connections to provide work for the associates below him. The paralegals generally supported a specific partner and the attorneys under him, though they could be used by anyone with a time-sensitive matter. My world was finally coming into focus.

The office dynamics also emerged. Susan, the paralegal I met briefly while I sat in on meetings during my summer internship two summers before, worked primarily for Eric and had been working with him for twenty years, beginning at his previous firm. It became very clear from the outset that she had her favorites, and she abhorred Jay, because of his cut-throat approach and his attitude, which she perceived as condescending to everyone below him, as well as what she saw as his moral hypocrisy. The associate one year my senior, Chad, also worked primarily with Eric, but also did work for the other partner and for Jay, the most senior associate.

The new actors had been introduced and all seemed pleasant enough, and my place in this universe was clear, though how I could possibly succeed was not. I entered this scheme as the lowest man on the totem pole, working primarily under Eric but remaining at the disposal of anyone who needed low-level assistance.

Beyond that first day of introductions, the language they all spoke was not the one I had spent the last few months learning. "Seven" was not an answer anyone would recognize, and no one was proud of me for arriving on time or packing a nutritious lunch. I knew absolutely nothing about what I would be doing. I transitioned away from my rehabilitation mindset to the other world I knew. Accustomed to the teaching methods of school, I waited for the moment when someone would stand before me and instruct me in precise detail what I needed to do.

This rarely materialized, though I did soon discover when my learning opportunities would present themselves.

Eric emphasized in my first meeting with him that Susan would be my greatest resource since, with her experience, she understood far more than I would for a while. He also positioned me so that I was working with Chad on most deals, making the two of them my de facto instructors and my most consistent contacts at the firm. I would be groping around in the dark, lost in this almost infinite world of legal knowledge, which was an extremely unsettling proposition, but I would have two guides, people who would mentor me along while doubling as my amateur psychologists.

Eric worked primarily as lender's counsel, drawing up loan documents that would set forth the terms of the loan and provide the lender with an interest in the property that was being purchased with the loan. Significant amounts of due diligence were necessary before a bank would lend a borrower money to purchase land.

He began to pair me with Susan and Chad to do this analysis, which usually took the form of title and survey work for these deals. Since the title insurance company was, for a fee, insuring that the report it provided listed all legal encumbrances on the land, we had to carefully review the report to make sure the land met all of the lender's requirements to serve as collateral and to make sure that the title company would protect our client if any problems did occur. We would sit at a large conference table, and they would flip through the Lender's Title Report to confirm that there were no unsuitable exemptions from the report's coverage and that we had the necessary endorsements from the title company protecting the lender in the state in which the property was located. Chad patiently explained to me why each endorsement was necessary in a particular instance, and we then confirmed that the legal description on the title report matched the survey done of the covered property to make sure the land for which the lender sought protection was the land covered by the title report.

"Beginning at a metal stake on the northeast corner of the intersection of Peachtree Road and Willow Street...," Susan would read as my finger found the point and began tracking the lines around the survey, confirming that no plot was missing from the report while I noted any irregularities in the legal description in pencil to have the title company correct. My life direction began at a metal stake at the intersection of two roads.

Thus, my days initially consisted of learning the basic grammar of this new world. Chad and Susan worked diligently with me on the title and survey work, Chad tasked with training me so that he could move on to more difficult assignments while I took his place doing the rudimentary due diligence. And it stuck. Owners' Policies, Lenders' Policies, Endorsements, ALTA surveys--the nouns began to come into focus. The nuances were sure to follow.

There was an added bonus to the instruction. Because of the frequency of my work with them and their friendliness and willingness to accommodate me on the team, I quickly came to see the two of them as my good friends in the office. I dropped in on their offices, which were situated next to one another, when I grew antsy to chat in my native tongue, and I began to get to know them better.

Susan usually seemed to welcome my intrusions, unless she was slammed with work, which she signaled with a brisk, "I can't talk today," at my pause in front of her office door. On most days, though, she greeted me warmly and chatted openly. During our conversations, I came to know her as a politically left-leaning idealist who had become a paralegal and ended up in Corporate America, though her disdain for the corporate elites all around us was never clearer than when, voice full of venom, she labeled one of them a "Republican." Her stories were lively, her laugh was quick and liberally dispensed among friends, though she kept her circle of friends tight, and her tone turned caustic when discussing individuals who drew her ire. She had certainly taken a far more roundabout journey to the firm than my straightforward jump from school, and she was the first to open my eyes, however briefly, to the idea that one could live a life not pre-planned since high school. She had married when she was younger but divorced many years ago. Her dog, Jake, was prominently featured in several pictures around her office and was a frequent topic of conversation when we spoke. She was a teacher, a friend, and an escape from my ongoing daily confrontation with confusion.

Chad joined her in these roles. When I was in Chad's office and his daily lesson concluded, I tried to engage him in conversations about other subjects. I learned that he grew up in a small mining town in Pennsylvania and, when I questioned him about the various diplomas on the wall, I discovered that he had graduated from UVA in 2000, one year ahead of me. Unlike me, he worked hard the entire time he was there, and, after graduation, he attended Vanderbilt for law school. Upon graduating from Vanderbilt, he took a job at another big law firm in the city, which was known as a family-friendly firm, with his wife, Valerie. Once he arrived there, he found himself working predominantly for a partner with whom he did not get along, and lateralled from that firm to our firm when Eric was searching for associate help in my absence due to their sudden influx of work. He was a reserved and diligent worker in a business where most people ventured opinions on everything and looked to avoid the most difficult assignments, and his Northern political sensibilities left him biting his tongue in any office political discussions. He and Susan were two of the few people who appeared genuinely unconcerned about the firm's prestigious reputation.

Since neither Chad nor Susan followed the political leanings of most of our office peers and their worldviews differed so markedly from most of the others around me, I came to see them as an isolated group within the office. In addition to working with them on assignments, I found myself associating with them socially as well. The contrasting personalities of straight-laced Chad and Susan's free-spirited approach led to an interesting group dynamic, but one that still presented a united front against the social and administrative pressures of the office. I soon found myself looking forward to our lunch outings, which were the highlight of my otherwise overwhelming days. My survival often became enjoyable thanks to their presence.

On the weekends, though my address had changed, many of my relationship dynamics had not. Mom still regularly returned to check on me to make sure I was able to handle everything on my own, and she generally brought food that I could freeze and reheat during the week, since I was a terrible cook. Her first trip found me tired but generally in good spirits, though I still was not putting on weight.

She could not do anything about this problem except encourage me to eat more. Instead, she helped me to tackle a more fixable problem, my transportation issues. During subsequent trips in January, she took me to look at cars, the newest item that dominated my thoughts. I looked at a Toyota 4Runner, a car I had dreamed of since I was in college, but I knew its size and available features were not what I needed, especially in light of the large monthly car payment it would require. It had been a dream I chose arbitrarily and, faced with my reality, I chose to eschew this option for something more practical.

I looked at the slightly smaller Highlander, which seemed to be a suitable alternative. Still, after considering all of the safety reviews of the cars in my price range and basing my decision predominantly on this factor, we journeyed to a nearby Subaru store and I test drove a 2004 Subaru Forrester, a car equipped with an armada of airbags and assorted other safety features. It was a vehicle my friends would later term "The Pillow Car" and would adequately protect someone who had recently invested considerable amounts of time and money in retaining a pulse. The car handled well, accelerated quickly, and would be at my disposal whenever I wished to drive to any location I so desired. A weekend snowstorm closed the dealership and delayed the purchase for a week; a snowstorm in Atlanta delayed my far more practical dream. But this time the weather created only a temporary delay, and when Mom and I returned the following week, she engaged in the expected horse-trading talk with our Samoan salesman. At the end of the successful negotiations and excited by the first major purchase of my life, I left with my car.

My capacity for newfound freedom aside, I found myself as constrained now by an endless list of tasks to accomplish as I had been before. My weekdays were not relaxing, despite the fact I was still working only part time. I no longer had to wait for the bus, which saved almost an hour each day. Even when I drove to work around ten and I left for home at three, though, I was absolutely exhausted. Furthermore, I seldom obeyed my restricted work schedule, arriving earlier than scheduled and leaving later in my attempt to prove I was a team player who could be relied on, even when Eric encouraged me to go home as scheduled. I still remembered my vow from the hospital room. I would not waste this chance, no matter how willing my body was to quit.

The doctors had warned me of the fatigue problem. My brain had to take the long route to avoid damaged areas when processing information and this required more energy, they told me, trying to boil complex neurologic explanations down to the most basic elements. My need for sleep would gradually diminish, though never completely, but initially I would need to get at least ten hours of sleep a night to recharge.

Their advice was not helpful. Medical science decided long ago that I was to die, and I defied it then. My obstinacy returned. I had too much to do to close my eyes and pretend everything was okay. Upon returning home from work, I knew I could not relax. I recognized that I still needed to improve physically to get all the way back but was unaware of how glaringly deficient my cognitive abilities still were. Every afternoon I ran for miles on the treadmill or lifted weights in my apartment complex's small gym, and then I grabbed a shower and tried to fade to sleep with Man on Fire playing in the background. But my eyes would not stay closed, even during the assigned period of rest, and I watched three become three-fifteen.

There was more to do, and my mind was working overtime, its limited efficiency leaving it to overheat at night, a week of sleep narrowly cresting my ten hour daily requirement. Even working part time, there was no time to focus on the trivial and expand my social circle beyond Chad and Susan at work. With all my efforts directed toward fixing the physical problems, there was little energy left for anything else. I saw these days as one final push to complete the physical repairs, believing my mind would fix itself soon.

{chapter 9}

My spare time, and even some of my time at the office, was dedicated to completing my reclamation project. I sat in my office many days and squeezed a spring-loaded gripping device with my left hand to regain strength and dexterity while I read the day's documents.

Aside from my physical deficiencies, I also found myself faced with a world in which I was a known commodity, but I was without reciprocal knowledge of my surroundings. I longed to remedy this information discrepancy by recapturing the experiences I had forgotten. My interactions with Amy, somewhat limited by distance and our respective obligations of school and work, moved to second priority as my quest for identity became all-encompassing.

My daily exposure to the office setting seemed to trigger random recollections of the summer prior to my wreck, a period for which I thought I had few if any remaining memories. In one particular memory, I could see an image of a woman, nothing more, and I began to ask Susan if she could tell who this was. Susan said it sounded like one of the second year law students, named Stacy, who had summered at the firm while I was studying for the bar. After asking around, I obtained her email address, and I sent her a simple email:

"Hi. My name is Neil Ligon. I believe we met last summer. I do not remember much from that time. Did we know each other then? I apologize if I am mistaken."

She emailed back and told me that we had in fact hung out fairly frequently the previous summer. My investigation into my past began in earnest, and emails to Stacy frequently followed my daily emails to Amy. I longed to know about me from the summer before, a period for which Amy's memory was limited by her geographic absence from Atlanta, and Stacy was a perfect conduit for this information. She would become the supplier of my recent past.

Memories did not come flooding back, but sporadically and randomly trickled in, in the form of incoherent images I could not understand. The image of Stacy looking back at me from a few feet away persisted, and I became uneasy about what it meant. Other memories stayed just beyond my grasp, and I knew more had occurred than what my mind could access.

I wrote the next email, knowing just how uncomfortable a position even asking the question put both of us in.

"I apologize if this comes off as presumptuous, and I do not mean it to be insulting in any way. However, I feel like there is something else going on here, and I just need some clarification. Did we ever hook up?"

Her response was curt. It was not a conversation she was comfortable having via email, but she would be in Atlanta in two weekends, and we planned to meet and talk then.

With the investigation suspended, I could think of little else. Impatient as to what this meant and unwilling to wait the requested time, I used my frequently ill-advised sense of humor to attempt further investigation.

"I am not going to owe child support, am I?" I callously joked.

She dismissed this as impossible.

We arranged a meeting time two weekends later, but I failed to disguise my curiosity in my emails. Finally, she acquiesced and provided me with much of the information I desired prior to our meeting.

"The summer of your wreck, we were good friends and we did frequently hang out. We were somewhat flirty on occasion but nothing that others would have picked up on. We both played on the firm's softball team, we hung out at parties at Todd's house, and we went to the movies together. We did hook up. Of the two times we did, we were both drunk the first time, and only you were the second time. We never slept together, though our interactions were not PG."

After the build-up that led to this email, I was not completely surprised by the revelation, though it remained disconcerting for me, considering I did not remember these events at all, and I had been cheating on the woman who had stayed by my side throughout the entire wreck and who remained my girlfriend. I was beginning to see that the life for which I yearned was not as pristine and free of concerns as I had once imagined. The man that I chased was immature and flawed. I did not pause to consider this and concerned myself only with juggling my desire to know more with a wish that Amy learn nothing else.

Stacy's words had not triggered a flood of images, or even a vague understanding of what she was talking about. This wasn't her jogging my memory. She was providing the only evidence I had of this time. I knew her to be an honest narrator, one I could trust implicitly, because…because I had no choice. It appeared that she had been honest with me before, and I thought it unlikely that she intended to deceive me, since she had willingly shared uncomfortable revelations in her emails thus far. Nevertheless, I knew that I would never be able to dispute anything she said.

The research phase of my recovery had begun, and with third parties feeding me memories, I began to think about this stage of my life, these moments of which I had no memory, in the same manner as they were told to me—in the third person. I had lost my connection with a past that I no longer recalled, and she who told the stories was a twenty-three year old historian, stoic and unaffected as an omniscient narrator moving forward a book that I skimmed to finish quickly.

The day arrived, and I travelled to hear the next installment of my life story. Stacy arranged to meet me at a coffee house in Little Five Points. I arrived early, fearful I would not be able to recognize her, and hoping to put the onus on her to find me. When she walked into the coffee house, I was able to identify her from the image I remembered, and I waved her over.

After the awkward handshake, we stood in line together. Our physical proximity did not indicate a personal connection, and our stances were wary. I purchased a pastry, since I did not drink coffee, and we returned to our table with our orders, where we sat and attempted conventional small talk, but the discomfort was palpable. I could see in her eyes that she knew me. There was an entire history in her head to which I would never be privy, and I looked out onto someone I knew only from a few random images and our recent emails. Her hesitations and her discomfort were not momentarily relevant to the narrative that I sat here hoping to piece together, so I did not notice if they were present or not. Still focused on how to handle a problem customarily relegated to Hollywood stories, I pushed ahead. The topic of my memory came up.

"I really don't remember much at all from that summer," I confessed. "I remember taking the bar, but that is about it. When you walked in, I recognized you, but I have images of you in my head, nothing more."

She suffered the blow nobly. "I know you've been through a lot, and when I heard about your wreck, I had a feeling you wouldn't remember me. I really just want to resume our friendship from last summer."

Since I intended to resume my past, I quickly accepted her offer. This portion of my return was already appearing to move forward surprisingly quickly. I finished my Danish, and after a brief hug and assurances of continued email correspondence, we left the store and got into our respective cars. My documentarian lived, and Amy would not need to know.

Stacy emailed again a few weeks later to let me know she was coming to town with another third year law student, Troy. I knew the guy who accompanied her far better than I knew her. Troy was a Vanderbilt law student a year behind me in school, he had summered with me when he was a first year law student the two summers before, and he had also worked with Stacy the following summer. They were coming to Atlanta to see one of Troy's favorite bands play. Stacy served as a freelance music critic who had been picked up by a number of publications in the past and was also interested in watching the band, so Troy swung through Athens to pick her up on his way in from Nashville. Troy's girlfriend, with whom he was moving to a different city after his graduation, despite my law firm's most ardent attempts to convince him to move to Atlanta, joined them as well.

Once they arrived in Atlanta, they came by my apartment and offered me a ride on their way to the venue in the Highlands, and we talked during the ride to the bar where the band was playing. I probed their memories, trying to gain additional insights without being too obvious as to my purpose. Upon our arrival, we all grabbed beers, which I was now authorized to drink. Mom, terrified at the prospect of me returning to the mass consumption that had plagued much of my recent past, warned me to limit my consumption to one or two, but I was not chaperoned and did not heed this advice.

While we watched the band, I drank liberally for me but not in an amount sufficient to alarm my companions. After about four beers, the music liberated me, and I began the white boy head bob and shoulder shrug that I spent much of my collegiate life cultivating. I brushed up against Stacy and unconsciously slid my hand into hers as the band continued on stage. The offer was not spurned, and my hand remained there for the rest of the song, me entirely oblivious to what I had set in motion.

After the opening band they had come to see completed their set, we stayed for most of the next band's set before departing for a nearby all-night diner. We sat and talked while tossing down greasy diner food. I listened to Troy explain how he had met his girlfriend and heard about the job he had taken in Charlotte. Troy and Stacy talked about the band and finishing up school. The topic turned to me, or perhaps I turned it to me. Surrounded by surefire successes and beginning to sense my intellectual inferiority, my stories dwelt in the superlative. They were to possess the first edition of a tale I would spend the next five years trying to refine.

"I was supposed to die," I told my captive audience, my voice remaining even to reinforce my emotional resilience. "During the car's rolls down the hill, my brain sheared against my skull and it scabbed over and it was only recently that the scabs were reabsorbed."

Forks discontinued their clatter against their respective plates.

"They had to rebuild my face with titanium plates, one they inserted above my left eye and one below my right eye, which they added by pulling my right eyelid out and sliding the plate into place through my eye socket." My hands directed everyone visually to the accompanying area on my face.

"No one was supposed to recover like I have—my progress is so remarkable that neurologists want to study me," I exaggerated, "but I don't have the time, since my job at the firm keeps me so busy. I'm really trying to put it all behind me and get on with my life anyway."

They nodded sympathetically. Even as we left the diner and finished the drive back to my apartment, my epic story continued. Finally, as we reached the last stop sign prior to our arrival at my residence, I wound it down.

{the detours}

They had heard the story, with all of its dramatic flourishes, not yet polished by repeated recitals, and I suspect they already understood what had happened better than I did. I would imagine they could hear my voice straining even before I was aware of the underlying tension. Still, I don't know if they could identify my desperate need for details to populate my description or if their attentions were effectively redirected by my hands' movements towards the sites of the trauma.

Whether or not they understood precisely what I searched for, they had to know that my identity was now based on this one event, and that nothing else would matter to me for a while. But they would never understand what I went through, no matter how much I wrestled with the words, tried to describe every detail with painstaking clarity, and infused each syllable with the raw emotion of someone shaped by an instant. That moment had made me but had not lent me even one detail I could claim as my own, and much of the recovery was hidden from view as well.

In truth, the story I recited to them was a compilation of police and hospital reports and inadmissible third party testimony. The feel of the rain as it splashed through the broken window onto my battered face, the pain of the seatbelt still digging into my chest even after the car's final roll, the smell of the wet earth permeating the vehicle—all these details were gone. I could not effectively describe something that I didn't myself know. I was left with only flickering memories of the monumental obstacles this event had caused, beginning in the Augusta hospital. The event that owned me would never be mine.

I bid them goodnight, told them to keep in touch, and walked inside.

It had finally begun. I had unwittingly started the task of building my own history, even while I lacked much of the necessary information, intent on being able to display this compilation as an apology. My more distant past remained as shrouded as it had before, but I had learned some of the boundaries of my fight. I remembered Troy, no matter how vaguely, from the summer we worked together, which indicated that much of the incompleteness of my memory was restricted to the summer preceding my wreck, a limited period I could work around. I reminded myself that it could have been worse.

{chapter 10}

My progress toward recovery was measurable. I quilted my past together, most days adding little pieces from hundreds of sources, until it began to resemble what everyone else's looked like. At work I felt stronger and stronger and, with the daily aid of countless gallons of caffeinated Coca-Cola products, dispensed from drink fountains in the recesses across from the partners' corner offices, I was making it through the day without showing outward signs of fatigue. I was ready to begin working full time. When I told Eric, he hid his doubts and simply requested that I have a doctor certify that I was ready for this.

So I returned to Augusta and asked one of the doctors involved in my recovery to sign a letter stating that I would be capable of working full time going forward. When I arrived, the doctor made a cursory inspection, asked me a couple of questions and then gave me a letter that left little doubt that I was capable of holding a job full-time. As she carefully crafted her note, the doctor must have known what neither Eric nor I could fully appreciate: there was no way to know precisely how my injury had impacted me or whether it would continue to affect my ability to perform a job about which she knew almost nothing. Regardless, I had a letter in hand that said little, but in my mind was the last bit of proof that everything was once again normal.

While I was there, I stopped by another location in Augusta to have my picture taken for the front cover of the regional rehabilitation magazine, which was doing a story about my accident and my subsequent recovery, another unprompted affirmation that I had made it back. I interviewed with the woman writing the story and confirmed the details of what had happened and told her about what I was presently doing in Atlanta. She thanked me and told me that the story would run in the Spring 2005 issue. I drove home to Atlanta a documented success.

I had left for Augusta that weekend to obtain proof that I was ok, but instead I was returning with a vaguely worded note and a sneaking suspicion, which I could not fully repress, that the definition of normal had changed permanently. Still, the documentation served its intended purpose, and when I presented it to Eric that Monday, he moved me to full time employment beginning the next week.

The weekend before my first full work week, Amy came to town to celebrate the promotion, and I took her to the nearby Maggiano's. I ordered a bottle of wine that looked expensive enough to drink on such an occasion, and after our glasses were full, I raised mine and toasted to us.

"I am finally the person you thought you were dating in law school. I'm going to make up for all of those months in the hospital. Everything is going to finally be okay."

I continued my explanation over the course of the evening. I omitted details that were problematic or unflattering. I excluded topics like the indiscretions known only to me. I ignored any doubts I had about our relationship. "We," "us," and "our" dominated the sentences. There would be no more bad times. The only obstacle to our happiness had been me, and I was finally "me" again. The team was finally whole. It was because of her that I had made it, and I would repay her for everything she had gone through.

She smiled at me from across the table, and as I inhaled seemingly unending amounts of food, I paused intermittently to reveal my plans for how everything would now occur. My ideas were the big dreams of a kid right out of law school, and my proposed career timeline allowed for no setbacks, since there was no reason to plan for something that would not occur. I felt certain that I had finally found my way back.

{chapter 11}

When I became a full-time employee, my pay increased, but it was at a tremendous personal cost. My employer began to expect more of me, more than I was confident I would be able to deliver. Title and survey work still dominated my daily routine, but I had graduated to new tasks, as well. I was also assigned to work under Jay, the senior associate, doing more complex work, though it was still the domain of young attorneys, creating documents from existing templates and revising them to include the desired terms. To do this, I needed an understanding of "boilerplate language," customarily found in all Georgia lending contracts, and what was deal-specific terminology that had to be changed each time. I had to understand more than nouns. I had to build sentences. I could not seem to grasp the concepts.

The pace was frenetic, as the Atlanta property values were soaring, and more and more entities were looking to buy land and buildings. I was entirely overwhelmed, and I did not know who to seek out with questions, as neither Susan nor Chad were working with me on these matters. I sat in my office paralyzed, almost in tears, my skyline view no longer providing the validation I so desperately needed.

I frantically flipped through the books on my shelf, thick treatises on Property Law, in the hopes of finding answers, but to no avail. Every couple of days, I would sit in a meeting and then return to my office with a specific assignment, nothing particularly complex even for a first year attorney, but still outside my realm of understanding.

Ideas were still dying too young. In the hospital, they had been stillborn of an amnesiac mother, witnessed only by random observers, painful memories to none. Gradually, though, they began to live long enough to haunt me, infant mortality fast becoming measurable. Sentences were lost for hours, only to show up again later in my mind's photo album. That was the reason I had told that story. That was the missing punch line. That was why I needed another signature block. My awareness of my incompleteness grew by the day.

I sought refuge in Susan and Chad's respective offices, and my daily tales of woe were sprinkled with moments of realization. I knew I was still forgetting a lot of things I needed to remember. I implemented my reintegration therapy strategies for coping with my spotty memory, but to no avail. Post-its littered my desk with reminders of what I needed, but they all too often failed to convey sufficient information to be of any use, and I spent much of my day trying to figure out to what they referred.

Additionally, the instruction Chad and Susan had in the past provided and continued to offer when I asked for help did not stay with me, and my learning curve was steep even for the most rudimentary processes. I struggled to learn the proper method to save a document onto our computer system, and I remained unsure of my abilities to even red-line documents in Microsoft Word, a straight-forward process with which to track changes made to the original document in the subsequent version.

These problems were beginning to surface even when I was part time, but they were not as readily identifiable due to my somewhat limited time in the office. Without the reprieve offered by a shortened workday, the Coca-Cola products no longer helped ward off my fatigue, and when combined with my frequent bouts of insomnia, my days became little more than laborious journeys into an enormous labyrinth of unintelligible legalese.

I was suddenly working for multiple people on several assignments at once, and though none of the assignments were particularly time-intensive, my inability to keep the details straight plagued me. The deals all seemed so similar. Eric would ask about how things were coming for a client, and I could not remember the parameters of the deal to which he was referring. Was that a sale-lease back deal? Or maybe that was the one where our client provided mezzanine financing? Wasn't it in Alabama? No, it had to be in Florida. I had not mastered the nuances of any of the concepts, and suddenly I was trying to fake my way through three different client assignments without a firm grasp of the details far any one of them. My mind dropped information with such rapidity that I could not even guess what I should have known.

"Did you remember to create the promissory notes for the revolving credit facility?"

I thought I did.

"Did you remember to use the ones we did for the lender's deal last November?"

I didn't know.

"Pull them up on the system and redline them to confirm that you used those, and send Susan your red-lines and your final version."

But I don't know how to do that, I silently screamed.

Figure it out, I thought. It couldn't be that hard. Didn't Susan show me how to do this yesterday? I hoped that once I pulled up the document, maybe it would all come back.

The document stared at me on my screen, and I slowly ran through the various menu options.

"Do you have those Promissory Notes for me on the deal we've been working on?" Susan's email inquired a few minutes later.

I tried to steady myself as I typed my reply. "I will have them for you soon."

I finally remembered that the redline function was found under the Tools menu, and I redlined the two notes against each other. The resulting document bled with red type. The two documents were entirely different. I had used the wrong template again. I raced to redo my work and sent the documents to Susan a couple of hours later.

This became my daily pattern. If I was lucky when I was confronted with an issue, I could seek out Chad, and soon he was doing my work as well as his own. On the occasions when neither he nor Susan were available to assist me, whoever I was working for suddenly became aware of my shortcomings. On one occasion, when I was working on an assignment for Sean, he stormed into my office and slammed down on my desk the document that I had finished for him earlier.

"What the hell is this? Did you incorporate any of the terms I gave you? This is unusable! Pay attention to what you're doing and clean this up right now! We don't have time for these kinds of mistakes," he yelled.

My days of pledging had long since passed, and I did not see it as my responsibility to suffer such indignities. I quickly pushed my chair back and staggered unevenly to my feet in the most threatening position I could muster, still unsure of my balance. My threatening posturing was as ineffectual as the rehab bully's had been.

In almost any other situation, my absurd insolence would have resulted in immediate termination, but with me, Sean didn't even notice. Instead, he merely looked at me without registering my intention and more calmly said, "I marked it up. Fix it."

My weekday routine did not vary too much from this regular pattern of intellectual rejection. I acquired the same paranoia that other first year associates did upon realizing how large a universe of knowledge they were already expected to possess. But the other first year associates began their tenure the prior September or October, and the people who would have been able to commiserate with me had I started with them were well past this stage in their careers. I was lost, alone and perpetually befuddled. I had fought so hard to return to an existence that I was finding to be miserable.

Susan and Chad did their best to console me, but I needed to start improving my work, and they both knew it. My emails to Amy, Stacy and anyone else who would correspond with me shared the same theme: I was certain to be fired, though I did not know when. I knew my employer would take my new identity if it saw the need to do so.

Any day in which I was without work for any period of time was a sign that they would terminate me the following day. Amy spent her emails trying to reassure me or distract me by discussing the coming activities we had planned. Any evening that Mom called to check on me, she was greeted by my familiar moaning about how I was about to be fired.

"Relax and do your best," she responded. "That is all you can do. Get your sleep so you're fresh for work in the morning. I'm sure you're doing fine."

Every day I returned to work—a pink slip never awaited my arrival. The grandiose visions of who I was to be vanished. Excellence was no longer a goal. Instead, survival became the new aspiration. My new goal was simply to maintain my position until the end of the summer interns' tenure, a period which stretched from mid-May to the end of July.

{chapter 12}

The summer associate program was designed to sell an image of opportunity and prestige to a group of law students whose grades and interviewing skills marked them as intellectually gifted, hardworking individuals capable of successfully traversing the political world of business relations. I had once been one of them.

The new chosen assisted with some of the projects, mostly doing necessary legal research or, on occasion and under close supervision, drafting specific rudimentary documents for a transactional deal. They silently sat in on conference calls with clients or observed team meetings discussing the status of different deals or cases. Each department vied against one another for the talent, though the first objective remained convincing these students to join the firm, and only then did each group's managing partner concern himself or herself about which individuals they could persuade to join their cause. All the while, the attorneys attempted to inconspicuously complete their work, to avoid burdening the summer interns with the knowledge that the large paycheck that awaited them necessitated sizeable quantities of hard work.

I was hardly an exemplary model of an associate, but I was close in age with the individuals who joined us, so I attended as many of the extracurricular events as I could. Such events provided an opportunity to socialize with people, something my prior schedule and absence of friends had not allowed outside of my time with Susan, Chad and his wife, Valerie.

Amy arrived two weeks after the first summer associates, and I suddenly found myself with a live-in girlfriend and awash with social opportunities. Amy joined us as we battled for intellectual supremacy during team trivia at The Dark Horse bar in the Highlands. I stood in the rain with Chad and a few willing summers at Music Midtown to watch one of my favorite groups ever, Public Enemy, which I memorialized with a black t-shirt on Irwin Myers' dime. And I made myself available whenever they needed another associate to balance out the numbers. I was acting as if I were still one of the interns, when, in fact, my role had changed completely. My gifts had been explored and my promise found wanting. To my employer, I was now one of the conquered, measured not by hypothetical tomorrows but by very real todays. I sensed this fact, even while I did not directly confront it, and I tried unsuccessfully to hide the paranoia that I was soon to be fired. I surreptitiously worked as much as possible when I could find people willing to provide me with work to do. My fear of termination did not dissipate, but I now had additional outlets for whatever remained of my energies. My spare time was no longer simply working out and trying to sleep.

Amy and I went out with the real estate department for dinners to help seduce the summers with promises of material success. My once abundant confidence was shaken, and social encounters with the summer interns, a self-assured group who occupied a seat in which I only recently sat, left me scared and stumbling over my words, much like my office encounters with my superiors usually did. Still, intramurals promised socializing without talking, awkwardness disguised by silence, and when we played on the work softball team, I felt that I might have found an escape that, though not perfect, I desperately desired. Our first time out, the self-assured associates and other attorneys described their talents to a receptive audience, ensuring their positioning at the front of the lineup. Without such a ringing endorsement from me, they chose to hit both Amy and me at the bottom of the order. As I stepped into the batter's box, the outfielders moved back in anticipation of a towering drive.

Instead, I looped a topspin liner a few feet over the bag at second; it dropped in safely and slowly rolled to the center fielder, who charged in to pick it up. I stood on first, relieved—mediocrity was the best I could have hoped for. Amy followed, and her five-foot-four stature drew the fielders in. The mammoth drive that followed easily cleared the left fielder's head and scored us both while the fielders chased down the rolling ball, which continued on unimpeded by fences. My coworkers, who now possessed situational evidence supporting my claim that Amy had played catcher at Columbia, batted Amy clean-up or fifth whenever she joined me thereafter, and I nosed my way up the lineup with my unspectacular series of singles.

Though I looked forward to the game itself, the competitive jitters that always preceded it limited my enjoyment. I simply could not free myself of expectations that I alone was creating. As each game would draw to a close, feeling more secure in the decreasing likelihood that I would make the mistake that would cost our team the win, I began to relax and listened in on stories reminiscent of my law school days that the summers discussed with the other attorneys.

But I didn't fit in, and that became clear to me early in the season. I wasn't a very good softball player, but I knew I never had been. Yet I also no longer had stories of drunken idiocy like the interns did, nor did I know who was playing the local music venue, the Tabernacle, that night, like many of my fellow associates did. I looked on at the events that transpired in front of me, and I knew I was merely a voyeur. I tried to recall my days spent there only two years before, but my attempts to channel the law school persona about which I had heard rang hollow—like the rehab biker's attempts to be intimidating. I wasn't that guy anymore. But now I was getting the sneaking suspicion I hadn't ever been him.

{it looked familiar}

As I spiraled inward, outward happenings escaped my notice. Amy's presence in my Atlanta life was because of an internship she'd taken at the Atlanta Solicitor's Office so she could live with me. Because her position was unpaid, her schedule was pretty open. Mine, on the other hand, was perpetually busy. Not only was I in the midst of an unrelenting identity crisis, but I was also embarrassingly inept at balancing my company-sponsored social life and my work schedule, even though the work assigned to me remained somewhat limited in its quantity. The summers had comparable skill sets to me, and some of the more basic work previously assigned to me was now passed off to them, which, naturally, exacerbated my certainty that I was soon to be fired.

My perpetual angst and the complete lack of a social life outside firm events meant that Amy was in Atlanta, knew no one else here, was meeting no one new and, on the rare occasion that I returned home at a normal hour with enough energy to be even mildly social, had to spend the whole time reassuring me that I wasn't going to be fired. I knew she wasn't happy, but I didn't know what to do about it, and after all of the nastiness she had gone through with me, I didn't think my present shortcomings were all that big a deal. Additionally, I was preoccupied with other aspects of my life and didn't have any energy left over to assign to our relationship. I thought I could take care of it later, once I got the other things straightened out.

In the weeks leading up to her arrival in Atlanta, I had decided I wanted a dog, and she agreed that dog ownership would be fun for the two of us. Once she joined me in Atlanta, I felt as if a common enterprise like caring for a dog would bring us closer and keep her distracted from our bigger problems, so we began our online search. I planned to save our relationship by enlarging our family without procreating.

We narrowed the list of acceptable breeds quickly. It couldn't get bigger than 50 pounds, since that was the weight limit for my apartment. It couldn't bark a lot. It couldn't shed too much. It had to be good with kids, because we didn't want to have to give the dog away if we had kids later on. I was unwilling to walk a dog that could be mistaken for a lap dog. With all of those prerequisites, our options were limited, and we quickly gravitated toward bulldogs or pugs. Pugs no longer remained part of the discussion when we learned of a potential issue with their eyes popping out. The decision had practically been made for us.

The French bulldog was the perfect size, but, in my personal opinion, was a bit too weird looking. This left English bulldogs, and our concerns that a mutt English bulldog cross would have a pit bull father made us wary of adopting a pound dog that looked like a bulldog. One day, Amy found a listing in the Atlanta Constitution Online classifieds for a puppy who had been returned after a few weeks, due to the adopting family's sudden move. She was a little older, around twelve weeks.

There were many English Bulldog breeders in the area because of the high density of University of Georgia alums and fans, but their asking prices were generally between $1200 and $1400. This breeder was willing to sell us the puppy for a mere $800, so we went out to look at the dog.

She was the single most adorable puppy I had ever seen, almost surreally so. She was white with black spots, similar to those of a Dalmatian, and her head was the same size as the rest of her body. Her butt was so narrow that it provided almost no anchor, and she looked like she was struggling to avoid falling forward. Amy and I returned home to discuss whether we wanted to get her, and by the next weekend, Amy borrowed $200 from her dad, and I provided the rest of the funds. I handed the breeder a check, and we had a hyperactive puppy we named Maggie at Amy's suggestion, since our new dog reminded her of the cartoon cow adorning Maggie Moo ice cream containers, with which she had grown up.

{it looked familiar}

With that, I had added another responsibility to my life, ignorant of the energy it would require but hopeful that the new addition would make the destination at which I had worked so hard to arrive more palatable. I had expended too much effort to achieve my goal to question its merits. Instead, I planned on adding accessories until it resembled what I might want.

Unlike Amy, I had never trained a puppy, and her patience with Maggie far exceeded my own. Maggie loved feet and had an obsession with shoes rivaling Eva Perone, leaving many of my shoes scarred with her teeth marks. Though my work shoes were kept out of her reach, my sandals lay about the apartment and were her frequent targets. My half-hearted attempts to scold her for chewing on them ended quickly when, with one of my size thirteen sandals in her mouth, she attempted to jump up onto the couch, barely getting the front half of her body up before taking a Charlie Chaplin-like fall to the floor on her back. I was a complete pushover and couldn't possibly muster further anger at our adorable puppy in those moments.

I knew my inability to properly discipline her was not helping her training, but I also came to the conclusion rather quickly that what Maggie possessed in cuteness, she lacked in intelligence. We tried to housebreak her, but she didn't seem to get it. We placed pee pads all over, in hopes that she would avoid peeing on the carpeting, and we vigilantly listened for her to bark to be taken out. But she barked at the door all of the time, and our efforts were generally rewarded by a playful panting and an otherwise blank look when we emerged outside.

On one occasion, after returning to the apartment from a walk, the sole purpose of which was for her to go to the bathroom, she made a beeline for the far corner and pooped. I was not impressed. She was shocked as the rolled up magazine in my hand smacked her on the nose while I yelled in dismay. She required two things I would willingly give only according to my schedule—energy and attention. She was no more a cure to the problems that plagued me than Amy was intended for the role of my career counselor.

She slept in the bed with Amy and me and, aside from her snoring, which I missed by falling into a deep sleep before any other inhabitants of the bed, she also had a habit of jumping off the bed onto the floor in the middle of the night. Upon arriving at floor level, she would change her mind and since she was too small to get back into the bed without assistance, she would stand on the floor whimpering until Amy picked her up and assisted in her ascent. I usually slept through it. I owned a dog, but I did not embrace the inconveniences. I was focused on me, blindly unaware that I did not evenly shoulder the responsibility for her.

Even my limited responsibilities for her daily care became a burden. I would come home from work tired and try to take her for a walk, intending to walk a mile lap through the neighborhoods behind our apartment. She would happily go along with me, abounding with energy, for about the first 300 feet. After that distance, the bulldog in her overpowered the puppy, and she would simply sit down.

"No!" I would yell at her while other people stared. "We're walking. You sat around all day. It is time for exercise."

I would shorten our distance and half-drag her through the neighborhoods until we returned, and I had to carry her up the stairs to my apartment, where her energy would once again return.

Even though she could be frustrating and frequently seemed like one more daily obligation, I needed her optimism, even if I could not afford the reasonable price she charged. She remained adorable even during moments of obstinacy and was so good-natured the rest of the time that she was one of my few daily bright spots. My frustration with her did not linger into my workday, though her non-judgmental acceptance sustained me. She stayed in the kitchen during the day, and when I would return home, she was the first to greet me, her clipped tail wagging so violently that it lifted her hind legs off the ground. Amy did her best to fake her enthusiasm about my return and listen to my daily tale of woe, but only Maggie could sell her excitement every day.

With Maggie in the apartment, she became the center of Amy's and my time together, and we were soon acting like a married couple with kids. When I was home, I played PlayStation to take the edge of the day off, decimating some team at NCAA Football with my ever more powerful UVA Cavaliers, willfully blind as to how dismissive this was to someone who had relocated predominantly to spend the summer with me.

Outside of the firm events we attended together, we met up with our law school friends down in Mobile for July Fourth weekend, we house-sat and took care of Susan's dog Jake while she visited Todd in Paris, and we ate occasional dinners with Chad and Valerie, but otherwise we kept to ourselves and played with Maggie at Piedmont Park. During one of our walks through the park, we ran into Jill, who I knew from law review at Tulane, and we exchanged information, but that was the extent of our social life unless Amy had a friend in town. I was isolated, and when she was with me, so was Amy. She was twenty-four and I turned twenty-six at the end of that summer.

As July drew to a close, the firing I knew to be a certainty never occurred, though I assumed they were waiting for the summer interns to leave before it happened. Amy's internship was over, and she was heading back to school the next weekend. Around ten at night on the Wednesday of her final week, we had a state of the union talk, in which we discussed the future. That night, she indicated that our visions of tomorrow no longer included the same elements.

"I can't live in Atlanta permanently."

It was such a simple sentence. It wasn't malicious; it was even spoken apologetically. It inferred a fact that had been self-evident for weeks. This wasn't working, and it was over.

I had not foreseen this possibility, and I was caught completely off guard by her declaration. We had a kid-approved dog together! I was working so hard to get my career back on track. The braces were gone, and I even had visible abs now. What else could she want from me? After all that we'd been through, why now? My life plan was going up in flames before my eyes.

"But I have to be here for my mom," I argued, since Mom lived two and a half hours away and had heart problems. I had once again missed the point. She didn't want to be persuaded. She wanted to be set free.

"I'm sorry, I can't live in this city," she quietly apologized.

"What does this mean?" I cautiously asked.

"I really don't know, Neil."

I suddenly realized it was over. My mouth made certain my conclusion was final.

"I guess there is no point in us continuing this if we won't end up in the same city, so I guess we are through."

She hesitated. I strained to hear her explanation of how we could remedy this problem, of how it wasn't over. But we had spent two and a half months together and had emerged with the passion of an old couple too tired for divorce. I was far too worried about myself to exert the necessary energy needed to make this work. Furthermore, the risk of having to find another job after a move was too much, especially considering how tenuous my present employment was and the high likelihood that I could not hold a job where people weren't willing to look the other way with respect to my mistakes.

She was tired of what we had become. She couldn't help but compare me to who she remembered from before, picking up on weaknesses that even I did not notice, and memories of our fun law school relationship made our present one even drearier. She understood what had been lost. She knew the person before the accident, a boy who still appeared strong and self-assured, and she knew who we had been together, kids sharing their school lives with one another. Despite all of my research into my past, I would never fully understand these things. The good things of the past were hers alone, since I remembered none of them. As for the present, I had not offered even a moment of the carefree fun a person in my position should have easily supplied since the day I left her house to check on Mom the previous August.

I wanted this relationship to work, but predominantly because I did not have the energy to start again. She had to know this. She had to be tired of babysitting her boyfriend. She surely wanted to be a girlfriend to someone she loved, not just a crutch. She had to see her Herculean efforts while I was in the hospitals as a sunk cost that would never pay dividends.

I don't know what she thought, because she wasn't going to beg for the privilege of more time in a broken relationship, and so she said little. Instead, she packed the rest of her stuff into her bags and, at eleven at night, grabbed Maggie's toys, bowls and other accessories and took them out to her car. I watched her disappear from the apartment carrying her stuff and return for Maggie. I was in complete shock by what had just occurred, but I believe the parting was civil, though I know Maggie looked more disappointed than Amy did as they walked out the door. I stood and watched the taillights disappear as they headed to her relatives' place in Tennessee.

One of the two constants in my life since the wreck would never again be present in a central role, and a dog that I had come to see as the embodiment of carefree hope would never greet me again at the door after another bad day at work. As I trudged back to the apartment, I felt like a fighter staggering to his corner at the end of a fight with too few rounds left to matter, knowing he simply could not land a punch. The bell signaled another round of being pummeled, nothing more.

I tried to lie down and get some sleep, since I had work the next day. But I was just in my empty bed staring at the ceiling, wide awake, considering the implications of what had just happened and waiting for my alarm to go off. The proclamation confidently made the previous spring at Maggiano's had proven entirely false. I was so broken that a woman who had once seen such potential when I was unable to walk no longer saw enough left in me that day to stick around.

I showered and threw on my work clothes at two in the morning and drove to the office. I deliberately strode from the elevator to my office and threw myself in my chair. I rotated around to face my wall of windows. Despite the hour, the outside of the skyscrapers remained lit. It was a spectacularly beautiful view. And it meant nothing. I turned to my computer screen and began typing an email that I thought might explain my outburst a few hours before.

"I cannot continue dating you, pretending that everything is fine when, at the end of the day, I know we cannot end up together. This is why I had to end it this evening when I learned you would never be willing to move to Atlanta. As horrible as tonight is, and the next weeks and months will be, it would be even more painful if we put it off until later, when nothing will change."

The words I typed were delusional lies. I had played a game of emotional chicken, and she hadn't flinched. Why hadn't she realized I was all bluster and simply called me on it? She had seen, from the inside, how much I was struggling to keep it together. Surely she knew she was in the superior negotiating position, and that I would willingly modify my unyielding stance, even without assurances of her final destination.

It never occurred to me to question what was really worth saving. I may have made the parting official, but in her mind, it was already done. She wanted to leave, not reconcile. I was once again the last one to know.

I fitfully slept in my chair until the sunrise illuminated my office. I still had my career to worry about, and in the fractured new sunlight, I cleaned up the surrounding paper as best I could and began working on the previous day's assignment.

{chapter 13}

She would change her mind, I told myself, if I could show her that I was still getting better. I would let my job describe me more fully; she would then return and add the finishing touches. I redirected all of my energy into my job and self-improvement. My weight dropped again. Since my wreck, I had not once been hungry, meaning that I had to schedule my meals to remember them, and I had begun to deviate from my schedule and skip meals in my haste to fix everything else that instant. I remained as ignorant as ever about what I was supposed to be doing at my job, but I kept hurriedly seeking the answers, hoping to figure things out with Chad and Susan's help. I knew I had to fight harder to become who I was destined to be, and the struggle would simply add character.

Unfortunately, my efforts did not bear the intended results. Chad and Susan's tutoring sessions did not appear enough to save me, and my daily grind was otherwise filled with unending aches and pains, which I fought to numb with an industrial-sized bottle of ibuprofen, and was punctuated by the departing shuffle of my coworkers, which signaled the end of my daily failures.

The deviations from my daily routine were the only thing that comforted me, so I actively sought them out. When a random day was slow enough that Chad and Susan were not overly busy, we found time to get lunch together. The conversations and sustenance at our lunch outings guaranteed the nourishment that my empty life and frozen dinners could not.

On those slow days, we gathered at the elevators and headed down to Susan's Mercedes, her one splurge in a life otherwise dominated by frugality, and we stylishly departed for Son's Place, a soul food restaurant in East Atlanta. The door opened, and a jovial "Welcome to Son's!" greeted us. They knew Susan on sight from her frequent visits over the years. Their delicious macaroni and cheese and collard greens were combined with the day's featured entrée, which we timed to ensure was fried chicken, meatloaf or pork chops, and I cleansed my palate with a tea so sweet it made my teeth hurt before devouring the blackberry cobbler or some other desert special that day.

Other days we would walk to the nearby Italian restaurant Baronda, where I could nosh on calamari and devour my mushroom pizza while we sat outside and talked about the office briefly before quashing that topic and moving on to more pleasant ones, such as Susan's search for her perfect long-haired hippy boyfriend or Chad's discussion of the ATP tour happenings.

Frequently, as the clock ran down and our departure back to the office drew near, the topics became philosophical discussions by individuals unfulfilled by the attained dream of career victory, and Susan wondered aloud whether there was something more to life than shuffling paper for Corporate America. Though I remained silent, I quickly dismissed this indictment of the arbitrary goal I had tasked myself with.

My evenings were no longer burdened with the early summer's companionship. Instead, their quiet was now marked by obsessive workouts, churning out sets of 250 crunches until they totaled 2000, running religiously on the treadmill and working to ensure my bench press weight exceeded my own in the hopes that fixing the fixable, my physique, would be enough to overcome the unrelenting reminders of my intellect's weakness.

Though I now focused exclusively on myself, I remained in contact with Amy, ostensibly as friends. I was aware that I still needed someone involved in my life to whom I could vocalize my fears in hopes that they would stop haunting me, but rarely did I take advantage of her confidence. Instead, Maggie remained the centerpiece of our talks.

"Maggie went swimming in the hot tub. When we got back to the house, I took her into the backyard to run around. When I showed her the hot tub, she stood there looking at it for a second, then dove in," the email explained, detailing the latest Maggie adventure. Her frequent emails almost always included pictures of Maggie, which she went out of her way to term "our dog," despite the absurdity of a collective ownership structure when our interaction was so limited.

I hoped that the casual banter would lead to a renewed interest, a less focused reminder of me and our time together would fan the sparks which still remained, ignorantly believing something still remained that could be salvaged and that a reminder of my issues could revive anything but regret over wasted time. Regardless, I was not to be the central character in these final shared experiences.

Only two weeks into her time in New Orleans, a tropical storm was brewing in the Caribbean, and she was only mildly concerned about its approach, since both of the hurricane warnings from the previous year had been non-events when the storm veered before landfall. Still, since she had already planned to visit her parents in New Jersey the next weekend, she decided to move up her trip by a couple of days. She boarded Maggie and grabbed a Wednesday flight out. The hurricane gathered force and began to strengthen from a Category 1 to a Category 3, and New Orleans remained among its potential destinations.

Hurricane Katrina made landfall on Monday, August 29, and unleashed unparalleled destruction on the city of New Orleans as the levies broke and the city flooded. Amy was safe with her parents in New Jersey, but Maggie was not. My once seemingly important job no longer mattered to me. I strained to hear news about this calamity and was deaf to my other obligations.

Amy and I communicated frequently as she called everyone she could to learn what had happened to the animals in the city. The veterinarians with whom she had spoken informed her that they had waited until the last possible moment to evacuate, but they eventually had to leave. They left the animals with as much food and water as they could, but no one was present in the city to care for them, and they could not tell her how the animals were doing.

I refreshed CNN.com a couple of times an hour and, as the documentaries later highlighted, the news was always grim. New Orleans was in ruins and floodwater covered huge swathes of the city and surrounding area. Shot after shot of rescue helicopters picking up people off of the rooftops of their submerged homes appeared.

There was no good news. People discharged guns at departing helicopters. There was mass looting. Some nursing home workers left elderly residents behind as they fled.

I tried to put my specific concerns in perspective. The carnage was unbearable to see, and the body count was certain to continue rising. Maggie was a dog, I told myself over and over, as I sat dazed in my office, refreshing my screen and emailing Amy. There were people who were dying in the city who needed help, and I began the grieving process, trying to remember that I had lost a pet that was no longer even mine, and everyone else had lost houses and loved ones, elements which defined their lives. Amy's emails remained optimistic that Maggie was ok.

"The facility is uptown, above where there is flooding," she explained. "It is a windowless building, so it had to withstand the winds."

But, as I told Chad, this was more willful blindness than it was realistic optimism. No one had been in the city to care for the animals since the day before the storm hit, and far more immediate concerns meant there was no timetable for when they would return.

Five days later, the veterinarians were allowed in. I cannot imagine what they saw, with one exception, something I imagined every day when I needed to feel better. Maggie was alive. In fact, she had eaten so much while she was there that she was heavier than she was when they had left her. I could see her stubby tail wagging emphatically when they opened the door and trudged in, fresh from witnessing the unspeakable horrors of the city outside. I knew that in that brief moment, they had been able to smile.

{chapter 14}

Hurricane Katrina impacted people across the nation, and it was no different in Atlanta. Chad's in-laws lived in Lake Charles, Louisiana, and Valerie had friends in the affected area, though her parents remained safe. Outside of major damage caused by falling trees to the surrounding homes, her parents' house remained fine, and they were safe but shaken. People around the office spent the week trying to sort through what had happened, but firm life went on.

As I tried to resume my normal routine, I felt pulled in another direction. I couldn't precisely pinpoint it, but my evenings frequently found me in a bar close to my apartment, downing a couple of cold ones while I devoured fried bar food. Nothing made much sense. I had virtually no friends, I knew my continued presence at the firm was a product of loyalty and nothing more, and I had no idea what I could do about any of my problems. Even with my horrendous diet and sporadic eating, my workouts had left me cut and physically stronger than I had been previously, but that didn't provide the solution for which I was searching. I was completely rudderless at a time when even a semblance of direction could have supplied temporary purpose.

To compound things, Stacy now worked with me. I was supposed to be the golden child from before the wreck, but after only a couple of weeks there, her work was already superior to my own. I didn't know how to do much at all, and I watched her handle with ease assignments that I still struggled to accurately complete. I was competing against her because she was present—in reality I was still competing against myself.

Why did everything have to be a competition with myself of old? I needed easy victories to restore my confidence, and that imagined me was unbeatable. That me was a product of inaccurate stories, with little basis in fact, coming together to describe someone who likely never existed, who I barely knew and who, from the sound of the disparate stories I was occasionally treated to, no one else knew as well as they had believed. I would never win this competition, but that didn't stop me from trying. I would earn what I had been given. I thought I could vanquish my demons with tireless effort.

Having my former pen pal in the office should have made this easier. I had described much of my struggle to her, and she had always offered to help in any way she could. Having a confidant, someone who would help me shoulder this load, was what I needed. But faced with the prospect of her intellectual superiority, my visits to her office were tinged with shame. Further compounding my inferiority complex, she had a seemingly unending line of social obligations, many of which stemmed from friendships arising during her time as a freelance music critic, a hobby that occupied much of her remaining free time. She would write about a performance and newspapers would publish her piece.

Even then, I knew it wasn't that easy, but it seemed as if when she tried, she succeeded. I would not go into her office to confess my jealousy, to talk about a longing to be more than I was then and would likely ever be, not only because it was inappropriate, but also because I was too embarrassed to admit any of this even to myself, much less to a peer. She had a more successful career as a hobby than I did as a job.

She suffered from the same insecurities that many other people did when they had just begun a new job and changed cities permanently, but I didn't see any of it, and the insecurities she did admit, I quickly forgot. I thought she was just trying to be empathetic while she witnessed me suffering. I saw someone who had always been successful and continued to be. I could ignore the vulnerability she flashed on occasion because it was usually so well hidden, while mine was perpetually on display. The possibility that she genuinely wished for a reciprocal friendship never occurred to me, even when she made this hope explicit.

Aside from Chad and Susan, she was my only friend in Atlanta, so my embarrassment did not dissuade me from stopping by her office frequently, but I stumbled over my banal statements, and I provided her none of the reassurances I actively sought from her, since I did not see how she would need them.

I talked incessantly, even when there was nothing left to say. I knew everyone, including me, was tired of my complaining. Mom begged for some positive news on our phone calls now. It was my burden, not everyone else's, and I was beginning to understand that people did not become friends because they wished for additional problems in their lives. It was supposed to be a symbiotic relationship, where both parties looked to one another for help. But I was too weak to even handle my own issues, and when I spoke or listened to people speak of other matters, I spent the entire time trying to repress the confession that I was miserable, as if I did not already wear it. Instead, I prattled on about the unimportant, still deaf to the words of my victim.

Day after day, I appeared in Stacy's doorway, looking the part I did not want to play, watching how inconvenient and disruptive my presence could be. When she looked up from her computer screen, still considering the language of a complex assignment she was expected to complete even while our amateur counseling sessions took place, I struggled to keep up with the conversation. I couldn't face it, so despite the close proximity of our offices, I resorted to email correspondence with some regularity, as it was an environment where I could collect my thoughts, smooth out any awkward wording and eliminate any unintentional innuendo. I knew everything would be ok, if only I had more time.

One day, I received an email from a concert promoter informing me that Weezer was playing the Gwinnett Arena and, since I had always wanted to see them, I forwarded it to Stacy to see if she would be interested. I knew Chad would probably not want to go, and I didn't know anyone else I could ask. My three person social circle left me with few options, and going it alone was never an option.

She agreed to join me, out of a sense of obligation, perhaps, or maybe because she mistakenly believed that the promise of a good concert outweighed any potential awkwardness that might occur. Or maybe she actually wanted to be friends, even when I didn't understand the concept. I was unconcerned with her motivation—instead, I grabbed two tickets, since the unending monotony of my existence was significantly more palatable when I found social activities to which I could look forward. The days preceding our event flew by, sprinkled with occasional lunches with Chad and Susan.

When the big day arrived, I packed my Public Enemy t-shirt, a black t-shirt that would help me avoid the black light, and the jeans and flip flops I was accustomed to wearing outside of the office. This escape to what I perceived as the critically accepted stylings of Weezer seemed to affirm my intellectual sophistication, and the Foo Fighters, the band formed by former Nirvana drummer Dave Grohl, were even opening for them.

Stacy and I left the office at a reasonable time, and she drove us to Gwinnett Arena. We had something to talk about, a mutual interest devoid of competition. She was my superior in the realm of music, but I was comfortable with this. We discussed the bands in depth, as I tried to tap into her extensive musical knowledge so I could accurately anticipate what I was about to see.

Upon arriving, we made our way to the floor, and the crowd's energy was electric as the Foo Fighters began their set and plowed through a few songs I recognized from the radio. I stood, feeling the music wash over me, and I felt invincible. Stacy danced in front of me, and I watched her move subtly with the music as if to let it pass by in the crowd. As I watched her sway, I confronted the physical draw but held myself back and let it pass with the floating notes. I was not as quick to dismiss my second reaction. Standing before me, I saw the memories of the days I wished for. She personified the success for which I was once destined, and I knew she could help me find that path once again. The Foo Fighters completed their set, and with the stadium noise limited to the surrounding crowd's chatter, individual voices were once again discernible. She was still facing the stage when I destroyed our friendship, isolated myself further, and embarked on another detour.

"This being friends thing is going to be hard," I told her.

She turned to face me and responded, not with a hasty retort to avoid exacerbating an awkward situation, but with a straightforwardness that left little room for debate. "No, it won't. I've had to get over you twice, and I'm not doing it again."

I mumbled an unintelligible response, as I felt my face flood with the red of mortification. Her gaze returned to the stage, and after a few dead minutes, Rivers Cuomo joined her there to end the cringe-inspiring silence that now hung in the air between us. I stood shell-shocked as the band wound its way through its newly released Make Believe album and finished their set with the old standard, "The Sweater Song."

With the concert over, we walked out to her car, and I smothered her with apologies the whole ride home.

"That was so inappropriate."

"God, I'm so sorry."

"That will never happen again, I promise. I got carried away with the music and the beer."

"I am such an ass."

"I am so sorry."

"I am so sorry."

She wanted the ordeal to be over, the discomfort to go away. She may not have known precisely what she wanted our interaction to look like, or perhaps she simply desired the stable friendship that I promised but failed to deliver. Most likely, I was not important enough to merit such intense deliberation, and getting me out of the car without further incident was the overriding goal.

"There is no need to apologize," she assured me, as I sat staring ahead at the red light that remained the final obstacle to our arrival at my place and my ability to escape the humiliation. "You didn't do anything wrong. We will sleep tonight off and everything will be fine tomorrow."

As I exited the car, I issued one final apology, and I climbed the stairs to my floor. The adrenaline raced through my veins in such quantities that I had to use both hands to steady their shaking during the key's approach to the lock. Finally, it slid into place and the door swung open. My two-bedroom apartment came into view. I walked to the bathroom and flipped on the light. My reflection stared back at me, its disappointment readily apparent, and I moved closer to inspect the image further. I looked the same as I had four hours before and quite similar to the guy I had spent most of my post-high school life being, even while this could not have been further from the truth. The scar on my cheek was beginning to fade, and I resembled the UVA kid who had ambled about Charlottesville with no pressing concerns and a lifetime ahead of me.

The right I landed staggered my reflection, and my hand began to throb.

"What the fuck is wrong with you?" I screamed at him. "Why can't you get this right? Just fucking fix it!"

I was too angry for tears. I stood before the old me, and I saw my greatest fears. There was no reset button. One day of my life would forever define me. I could make the scars disappear, but I was still a guy too bitter to have friends and too dumb to learn. I was trapped in a world that guaranteed failure. I couldn't do this anymore. I didn't know who I was, and I knew my once-promising future lay dead on a hill in Alabama.

I walked to the drawer and pulled out a knife. If I cut it along the vein, it would not clot. I carefully marked the target by running the blade slowly along my arm with enough pressure to leave a line that I could follow. The teenage angst fantasy ran through my head as I imagined the mourners comforting one another and once again speaking of me in glowing terms. And I saw Mom crying, wearing a look of indescribable pain. I placed the knife on the bathroom counter and picked up my Blackberry.

"Stacy, I need help," read the message, which I knew would be delivered instantly to her via her Blackberry.

{chapter 15}

Stacy compiled a list of facilities that could help me. There was to be yet another hospital in my future. I found the number for Peachford Hospital and dialed it.

"Yes, we can admit you if you come in," the receptionist explained, and she described for me where they were located. I packed a suitcase and headed to the facility, emailing work to tell them I would not be in that day.

When I arrived, I parked the car in the large but mostly empty lot and walked up the slight hill and through the automatic doors. I filled out the paperwork at the front, presented my insurance card and, after giving up my keys, and wallet, was led to the back. The room that the nurse led me to looked like an empty dorm room with two single beds, one on each wall, and I deposited my bag in the corner.

The escorting nurse followed me into the room and briefly summarized the daily routine, which involved group therapy sessions, individual sessions with a psychiatrist, constructive free time when we were allowed to go outside, optional AA and substance abuse meetings, regularly scheduled meals, and some free time we could allocate as we saw fit. I asked the nurse for paper and a pen before she left, and she returned with both, which I placed on top of my bag.

I returned to my bed, hoping this institution would provide the answers that the other hospitals could not. An orderly making her rounds summoned us to gather in the main room for the staff and the patients to introduce themselves. I looked around the room at my new cellmates. Everyone seemed pretty ordinary, with only a few exceptions. Many were present because of substance abuse issues, whether their treatment was court ordered or self-imposed. Everyone was there fighting against something that rendered them helpless.

I was allowed a phone call, and I called Mom to inform her of my newest location.

"Hi, Mom," I began, trying unsuccessfully to quell the panic in my voice. "I don't want you to worry, but I need you to know where I am. I checked myself into a psychiatric hospital."

"Relax. It's going to be okay. What is the name of the facility?" she asked, concern buried far too deep beneath layers of comfort to be noticed.

"Peachford Hospital. It's north of the city."

"Are you okay?"

"Nothing bad happened. I just panicked. I don't know what to do anymore. I'm only going to be here for a few days. I already feel better."

"It's going to be okay. So many people love you, and we are here for you. I'm proud of you for getting help. Listen to your doctors, and everything will be fine. Is there a number where I can reach you?"

I provided the information and explained the constraints on my ability to call out but freedom to receive calls of a limited duration.

"I am going to have Colin call you, because I know he will want to talk to you."

Our brief conversation ended, and I hung up, devastated at how the sickness was spreading across my life. My family now knew. The magazine article proclaiming me a success had been written too early. I knew the facts it had detailed had not been quite right, and I finally understood this had led them to the wrong conclusion. I was a failure. Part of me held out hope that it was temporary, but I could feel the doubt settling in. It was over a year later, and I wasn't better.

{chapter 16}

I found activities to keep me busy during my stay. I attended an AA meeting, and after listening to the group, I suddenly worried that I was an alcoholic, though many of the stories I heard reflected extreme manifestations of this behavior and relationships lost, neither of which I experienced due to my occasions of overconsumption.

When I met with the psychiatrist, I summed up my predicament succinctly.

"I had a severe traumatic brain injury. My memory doesn't work anymore, and I do not know how to cope with this. My life is a complete mess, and I have no idea what to do to fix it."

"Were you considering killing yourself?" he questioned as gently as the topic would allow.

"Yes, I checked in here because I was thinking about it."

"You were afraid you would go through with it?" he asked.

"I was, but I don't think I was actually willing to do it," I responded, already becoming exasperated. He was missing the point. My intentions the previous evening were wholly irrelevant to what I needed now. I needed him to fix me. His initial diagnosis was severe depression, and he put me on a formidable antidepressant immediately, which seemed to help right away, despite the fact the medication would not start working for a few days.

In between my scheduled events, I documented my thoughts in a yellow notebook before they could depart into the ether. I tried to control my fears by naming them.

The sound of my mom's voice finally brings the tears that have been hiding, I furiously scribbled onto the page. It is unspoken, but we both hear it clearly. I can't fix it. I don't even know what "it" is. What if they can't either? I'm back depending on others for things I cannot do. I've been five twice already. The third time brings a new level of powerless without the carefree innocence of the first.

But after two sessions with the psychiatrist and frequent entries onto my yellow tablet, my head began to clear, and I felt fixed and wished to resume my life. Still, even for individuals who voluntarily checked themselves in, the hospital had to observe each person for three days to determine that they were no longer a threat to themselves. Despite my awareness of the embarrassment awaiting me at the office, I itched to return to my life after the first two days. I had to remain for an additional day however, despite my pleas that such a delay might result in the termination of my employment. Regardless of the delays, the pills should take care of the unhappiness, I thought, and maybe they would calm me down enough that I could once again have normal friendships. The pills had to be the answer.

The psychiatrist and I had our last session, and though he expressed concern over my ability to handle everything that was in front of me, he admitted that I no longer posed a threat to myself and duly signed the discharge papers. He gave me the name of a psychologist with whom he advised I should meet and wrote a prescription for the anti-depressant I was taking, which he said I should continue to take until all of the pills were gone.

I signed the discharge forms, gathered all of my belongings at the front desk, and walked out the sliding doors I had tentatively entered three days before. I knew that I was about to experience months of uncomfortable social situations at the office, but I didn't have much choice. When I got into my car, I grabbed my cell phone from the glove compartment where I had left it and saw that there was a message waiting for me. It was Chad, and he was explaining to me that I would be living with them for the remainder of the week. It was not an invitation; it was more a friendly command. I called him back, and he detailed the offered accommodations with the zeal of a real estate agent.

"You may have noticed, but the basement bedroom has its own bathroom and shower. We keep the door to the downstairs closed, so you shouldn't hear us at all. It stays cool, which is nice this time of year, but we will leave extra blankets down on the bed in case it gets too cold."

"Is Valerie okay with this?" I asked. "I don't want to intrude."

"It's fine, it's fine. You won't be intruding. Valerie suggested this before I even asked her," he assured me. "You can join us for dinner after work in the evenings, too, and you can follow me into the office in the morning."

"Okay. I need to run home to pick up my clothes and take care of some things quickly, and I will give you a call to let you know I'm heading your way."

Chad was offering me an Atlanta family, and my acceptance of his offer was never in question. They had a German Shepherd-Chow mix named Peyton with whom I was familiar, and, when I arrived at their house a few hours later, Peyton greeted me with his usual energy, enthusiasm and goofy acceptance as Chad invited me in. No one grilled me about what had happened, and when I expressed my reservations about what people would say when I returned to work, Chad assured me it was nothing to worry about. The next morning, after a surprisingly peaceful night's sleep, I swallowed a miracle pill, grabbed a shower, threw on my work clothes and followed Chad in to the office.

Stacy had gone out of her way to make a peace offering after her email that gathered the information about psychiatric facilities. In the second email, she tried to even the information disparity between the two of us by detailing a great number of personal anecdotes and revealing many of her personal insecurities and the accompanying incidents that caused them throughout her life. I appreciated the insights, since the threat of mutually assured emotional destruction theoretically evened the playing field and provided me insights into a woman I did not know. No one else breathed a word about where I had been, with the exception of Susan, who asked if I was okay.

Midway through my day, Eric called me into his office. Grasping at straws, trying to reassure me that my latest issue was not a unique problem, he did his best to hide his discomfort with the topic at hand. I was nervous when I walked into his office, since I had no idea what he would say.

He opened with, "Are you doing okay?"

"Yes, I'm on medication, and I will be scheduling appointments with a therapist once a week," I cautiously responded.

He sensed my agitation and did his best to alleviate my concerns.

"Going to therapy is perfectly normal. Susan has been to a therapist before. If you need to see a therapist some mornings, let me know ahead of time that you will be in a little later. You don't need to notify anyone else. Send me an email, and I'll make sure it's taken care of."

The office-wide general silence and Eric's tolerant approach put me at ease, and I resumed my daily routine, thinking nothing much had changed.

{chapter 17}

Of course, everything had in fact changed. It had been over a year since my wreck, yet I had announced to everyone in the office that I still wasn't right. On its own, I doubted this would be sufficient grounds for termination, since few employers, even those with deep pockets, wanted to end up in court on the charge they fired someone due to health reasons, even if they would eventually win. Yet it added to the ever-growing number of examples of why my job performance was subpar.

The hum of Chad and Valerie's house kept the panic at bay for the first week. They went out of their way to accommodate me, and I fell into a routine with them. I helped walk and feed Peyton, and I ate dinner with them. But as much as they invited me in, I knew I was merely an observer intruding on their lives. Still, it was hard to pull myself away from the display, and I knew that this stability was what I wanted.

I was aware that on many occasions, they both felt overwhelmed with everything they had going on. However, in my eyes, though Valerie was also a busy attorney at another big law firm in the city, their running around generally had a purpose and because of this, felt finite to me, since it promised to end with the completion of the tasks at hand. My tasks were too numerous to ever finish. I wanted some limits on the efforts required of me, some semblance of certainty, and even their busy lives appeared to offer this, though they probably did not perceive their stresses to be as finite as I thought them to be.

The evening escape from the drain of the office was, if for only a few brief days, a stabilizing event. I had something outside of my job that I could look forward to. When the weekend arrived, I knew it was time to return to my apartment, so I thanked them profusely for their willingness to harbor a fugitive from reality, and I returned to my residence to face the music.

When I returned to my life, it was as empty as it had been before, and I begged for others to help me fill it. My family friend Alicia Stone began to come to Atlanta from Columbia; she was bored and seeking out alternative destinations to escape the town. Her visits meant a reprieve from my isolation, and Chad and Susan were no longer burdened with providing me with my sole social outlets. During Alicia's visits, she introduced me to some of her friends, and soon emails about her friend's weekend plans found their way into my inbox, as she proposed additional visits.

Even with offerings of borrowed social events trickling in, I felt isolated. I continued to feel lost at work and came to see myself as a caricature. I suspected that I was the slow cousin of the office, and I knew that I didn't follow the social and work protocols to which people assumed I would adhere. I laughed too loudly, smiled at inappropriate times, spoke on conference calls when my voice shouldn't have been heard, moped with such frequency that it made people nervous, and was always the weakest member of any team I was on.

Despite this or maybe because of it, I went out of my way to be nice to everyone, and I was trying so hard. I started to see the quiet pity in the eyes of people who didn't even know me particularly well when, unable to avoid a chance encounter with someone carrying the disease of failure, they ended up trapped in a hallway with me. Chad and Susan either didn't feel it or could mask it at all times, confirming them as my only safe daily personal interactions.

My workflow had slowed somewhat, as Stacy was now doing the majority of the work for Jay, though I did pick up basic assignments here and there from other sources. The ax that I lived in perpetual fear of never fell, and the last milestone of my employment goals arrived: I was invited to attend the first year retreat with the class below me and a few of the new laterals, which was to be held at the La Quinta Resort and Club in Palm Springs.

I was entirely shocked I had made it this long, and I struggled to figure out what this meant. I realized that on this occasion, why I was still there was not important, and I began preparing for the trip. It was a last reminder that we were still students pretending to be businessmen and businesswomen, so they scheduled some final classes in our respective areas of specialization during our stay and allowed us to perform a few skits, but we knew that after that weekend, we were expected to put aside such childish things.

In the weeks preceding our departure, our group gathered to prepare for our skit. We chose a script that Stacy had written spoofing America's Next Top Model, with contestants modeling stereotypical attire from the various offices, and ran through it a couple of times to ensure that we had the costume changes in order and the timing down. Stacy would MC it, and all we had to do was walk out on cue in the appropriate attire; I represented the Palo Alto office, and my costume involved glasses, hiked-up pants, and suspenders. I felt sure that I could play socially awkward, and the lack of speaking lines meant that I could manage to look stereotypically mathematically knowledgeable. I gathered all of my clothes, including my costume, collected my tennis racquets, and grabbed the ticket emailed to me and headed to the airport to fly to Palm Springs.

Once I landed in Palm Springs and made it to the resort, one of the staff handed me the itinerary and a welcome bag. I took the handouts and the gift bag and slinked to my room, committing another act of fraud. Unlike my hospital and outpatient admissions, where the paperwork I had presented to gain admission had described me with precision, the host of this weekend had been sloppy in his or her haste and had invited me by name, assuming that this moniker properly identified me as someone who would belong at such a prestigious retreat. But I wasn't like the other members of the group—those hardworking, intelligent first year lawyers primed for success. I wasn't the right age or on the right career trajectory to be there. I was using a fake ID.

There were training sessions I was required to attend relating to the real estate practice, but much of my time was free. For almost a week—with nominal obligations—I was in paradise on an all-expenses paid vacation I didn't deserve. I was terrified of being caught.

I knew this time served as a reprieve, not a pardon, from my career-ending sentence. I barely knew the people with whom I was on the trip, and I felt like an unwanted guest whenever I joined them, despite that everyone was friendly. I explained my wreck to anyone who would listen, since some may have wondered why I was on a trip reserved for their class and the accompanying laterals, but mostly to explain why I was struggling so badly, in case they'd heard the rumors indicating as much.

The relaxation everyone else embraced I found unsettling. I worried about messing up my part of our skit, missing the required classes, not fitting in, intruding on everyone else's plans and most of all, revealing my incompetence to people outside the Atlanta office who would demand action be taken to correct the situation. During the events, I said cringe-inducing things, like my statement attempting to ridicule the office stereotypes and my ability to summarize my identity in two sentences at our formal dinner.

"My name is Neil Ligon. I am an associate in the Atlanta office, and I like to go coon hunting," I announced to a room of horrified people.

I played tennis with Stacy and another woman who worked in the Atlanta office in the Corporate group, but I otherwise spent most of the time keeping to myself whenever possible. I sat in my room and played the game Memory, which I had packed, trying to retrain my brain to capture information. I ran the sections of the nearby golf course to continue my preparation for the 5K I was scheduled to run with Chad a couple of weeks after my return. I mindlessly worked through sets of pushups and crunches. I knew my present environment was another installment of what I couldn't have; I tried to block out the distractions and staid focused on the task at hand.

I didn't mess up my part in the skit, and thanks to the clever writing and some creative costumes, we won the competition with the other offices. We celebrated the victory with beers during the evening's outdoor festivities while everyone talked about their nervousness, the unseen mistakes they had made, and how tremendous the victory had been. I felt like part of the team.

"Yeah, I ended up in my black socks and work shoes at the end when I came out in my camo shorts and t-shirt. I was too buzzed to get my shoes off without falling over," I confessed to the group, laughing.

"Where did you get that costume, Kamran?" someone asked Kamran, referring to the traditional Indian garb he had donned for the mythical Bangalore office, which provided another moment of levity during the skit. The banter continued unabated, and for a few moments, all the social distinctions disappeared, and we became The Winning Team.

We returned to Atlanta with promises that we would all hang out together more frequently, but a busy work life limited these opportunities. Outside of hellos in passing, I rarely spoke with any of the people I met that weekend, and I resumed the usual grind.

Meanwhile, I had run out of arbitrary markers that I needed to make it to. I had survived my part-time stint, made it through the summer, and I had attended the first year associate training.

Maybe they weren't going to fire me. Maybe the frequent title and survey work I did was enough. I dutifully helped Susan with the files and found work coming across my desk frequently enough to calm my fears. The previously inescapable paranoia about losing my job began to lessen, if only slightly.

The awkwardness with Stacy did not follow my work paranoia's lead. I found myself tripping over my words with her and saying things I knew came off wrong. She would complement a shirt that I had bought the previous summer, while smiling a smile filled with knowledge, but my inquiries into the meaning of this would be quickly dismissed. The existence of formerly shared memories that now only she possessed was enough to make me afraid that every statement, every article of clothing, every joke I told had a meaning that I didn't understand.

I had tried to normalize everything, as had she, and it hadn't worked, I thought. Further efforts would be for naught, and I couldn't handle it anymore. One November day, after weeks of cringing in embarrassment at even the most innocuous of statements, my frustration finally spurred me to action. With the immaturity that dominated my interaction with her, coupled with a hereto unseen decisiveness, I walked into her office one afternoon and, with the speed of an auctioneer, blurted out, "I don't think I can talk with you anymore. Everything I say comes out wrong. I'm sorry."

She called after me as I turned heel and walked away, but any regret she may have had about the termination of our interaction ended with the shrill last sound of the final "l." Though my declaration had not changed our geographic proximity, Stacy worked primarily for Jay now, limiting our work interactions to once or twice a week. After my proclamation, I turned and walked out that afternoon and quietly shut my door. It would remain shut every day from then on to ensure my office isolation would only be interrupted with my permission. I would never have another extended conversation with Stacy again, despite the fact she continued to work two doors down from me. Our awkward friendship was over, and my inability to reconnect with someone once close to me served as a further daily reminder of my ineffectiveness in reclaiming even pieces of who I had been.

I had made myself my own island at work, except for my brief daily visits with Susan and Chad. But my life outside of work now provided the requisite social contact to sustain me in the short term, offering me more chances to reconnect with old friends and observe their seemingly linear trajectory. Kevin Butler announced he and Rachel were getting married in March, and he asked me to be an usher in his wedding. The emails flew around planning his bachelor party, and I discovered that I was more comfortable in my work seclusion, perusing the emails in my Hotmail inbox, than I had ever been associating with my coworkers.

I travelled to Tampa for another law school friend's wedding, where I had the opportunity to see friends from law school who had scattered as far as Texas. I met up with Jill, my friend from Tulane Law Review, at a local UVA game-watching bar and saw Virginia Tech pound our Cavaliers 52-14. Our conversations echoed the sentiment that rattled around the room after each score: our school was so far superior academically that we had to suffer through one football beat-down a year before spending the other 364 days enjoying the far greater prosperity our degree helped furnish. Quarantined at work, I was an unsuccessful elitist at home but, when accompanied by seemingly similar individuals, I could take a break from my self-pummeling and feel like I was fitting in.

{chapter 18}

I continued treading water at work, searching for human connections through electronic communications and sporadic after-work social events, and soon the holiday season was upon me, beginning with Thanksgiving, a government- and employer-mandated reprieve from work. I returned home to the safety of Aiken and had Thanksgiving dinner with Mom and Colin. My plate piled high with mashed potatoes, green bean casserole, stuffing and, my personal favorite, huge slices of a circular cranberry and Jell-O mold Mom had been making since we were kids, I gorged myself into my customary food coma. It was a lighthearted gathering, much as the holidays generally were with family, and Colin discussed medical school and Mom talked about the current goings on at her high school.

The planned celebration in Louisville, Kentucky, where my grandmother, uncle and cousins lived, was not going as smoothly. My Uncle Jim called with the bad news: Granny was in the hospital. When he had arrived to pick her up for their Thanksgiving gathering, she told him that she wasn't feeling well and that she was not going to attend. Within hours, she was in the hospital. She was stable, but not doing well. The news that trickled in throughout the weekend pointed to only one conclusion: she had begun an irreversible slide and it would not be long until she was no longer with us.

A somber mood hung over the rest of the weekend and all of our phones remained on, awaiting further news, though none came. Uneasily, we began the second phase of our Thanksgiving break, preparing for Mom's move to a house in a nearby golf community.

The house my brother and I were visiting, the one we helped Mom move out of, had been our home since we moved to Aiken when I was five. It hadn't been my first choice. I had fallen in love with another home that had a tree house situated in a large oak in the backyard; this fort was sizable enough to hold the army of new friends I was planning to make and stout enough to repel my brother and any of his friends from entry, should they choose to approach. Instead, my parents had chosen the house Mom was now vacating, a spacious ranch-style residence. My room was painted purple, no doubt at the request of its previous female occupant, and despite assurances this would change, I felt my newly assigned room to be unacceptably girly.

Still, the house had grown on me as I grew up in it. After our move down from Pennsylvania, my room lost its purple hue, replaced with white wallpaper featuring thin colorful stripes that ran vertically, interrupted mid-wall by a border of cartoon animals holding balloons, the rhinoceros looking on dejectedly at his deflated balloon, which hung from his horn. At one point, an eight-foot high basketball hoop had been attached to the side of the house, just above the garage, to ensure that my path to the pros would continue unimpeded. Only a re-staining of the wood above the garage masked the holes that were drilled to support the hoop during those years and the accompanying ball marks resulting from errant sky-hooks and heaved jump shots.

Later, aided by my dad's severance package from DuPont after they lost the Savannah River Site contract, a tennis court was installed, and I had hit hundreds of hoppers of serves in my backyard, the velocity beginning at the 30 mph mark and increasing with age until it crested 115 mph prior to my departure. I had sunk twenty-foot jumpers on the basket that was now suspended ten feet above the court, affixed to a pole in the middle of a near fence. I had spent countless hours mowing that enormous field, grasshoppers flying about me, as our riding mower sucked up the once unruly blades of various grasses. I had caught footballs lofted from friends there and had crushed hanging pitches from my brother over the far fence.

The following week, as we assisted Mom with the final preparations for her move to a more reasonably sized house, without the acres of grass she could no longer maintain without paid assistance, I felt unsettled. It was the practical thing to do, and I knew that. Before I departed, I took one last walk through my childhood home and the melancholy I experienced after my goodbye hung with me for the rest of my trip to Atlanta.

During this drive back to Atlanta, I came to the conclusion that I needed to go see my grandmother, though the likelihood of her recovery remained minute. The pull was unbearably strong, though the reasons behind it were only somewhat understandable. I had become aware over the previous year that my long-term memory was very spotty. Some events and people I remembered perfectly; others I could not remember at all.

But I still had many memories of my childhood visits with Granny and Papaw. I could readily recall pounding out note after note on the organ they had in the basement, much to the chagrin of everyone in the house. I remembered throwing the Nerf football with Colin in their front yard, trying to avoid the tree limbs with our arching passes. I could see myself perched on their pontoon boat, just inside the gate at Rough River, with my fishing pole in hand as we headed toward a promising spot to catch the big one that would make Papaw proud; all while Granny sipped on her Diet Coke. I could hear her voice encouraging Colin and me to "keep scratching," as we furiously rubbed the borrowed quarter against the scratch-off lottery tickets she placed before us, convinced that this one would be the $20 winner. Perhaps this was why I needed to see my grandmother, why I needed to see her to make a miraculous recovery.

That was certainly one element of why, upon my return to the office the next day, I walked into Eric's office and asked for the coming days off to go to Louisville to see her. But my haste in scheduling the flight out contained a desperation regarding the certainty of Granny's fate that should have now begun to temper. But it hadn't lessened at all, even after I chose my exit row seat and finalized my place on a flight that would certainly allow me to arrive in time to see her and to potentially watch her medically unlikely return from the brink.

The individuals who shared even pieces of my biological identity were beginning to disappear. Granny was my last remaining grandparent. Mom's mother lost a battle with cancer before I was born, and Mom's dad, who was in his fifties when Mom was born, died of natural causes when I was not even two. Her oldest brother, Felix, still lived in Chicago, but her middle brother passed away before I was born. On my dad's side, Papaw's smoking habit had resulted in a stroke, which he suffered while sitting at our kitchen table in Aiken when I was ten, and most of my life I remembered him in a wheelchair. He had survived my father, but he passed away while I was in college.

I could not tell how much I really remembered about my father, who passed away when I was fifteen. I could tell stories about events where he was present, but I could not recall participating in them. I remembered him without an accompanying soundtrack. I was there with him in a series of life events captured by stories that lost the humanizing details a dad would reveal to his son when he wasn't playing the role of a disciplinarian or universe stabilizer.

I no longer felt as if I knew him, and I had been hopeful that I could someday sit down with Granny and talk about him, hear about his childhood, listen to tales of his successes, and she would provide a window into the soul of a man I had always hoped to emulate. I had been so busy trying to get my life back together that, even as I saw some of the collateral damage to my long-term memory, I hadn't yet found the time to begin repairing it with supplemental anecdotes from others. This explained my panic on one level.

But my dad's brother, my Uncle Jim, lived in Louisville, and he could provide me most of these stories from my dad's childhood, and Mom could tell me stories from the rest of his life. The continued force of the emotions that I was feeling on this front remained illogical.

It finally occurred to me that this, too, was a product of my now uncertain past. In a world in which I could no longer access even the most indelible memories, I needed back-ups. People couldn't die. I was terrified of losing her, because it seemed as if my family members were all quietly disappearing, at first from my memory, and now suddenly from my life as well. I remembered Granny's voice today, but what about tomorrow? I could remember the nightly I-love-yous before Colin and I trekked down the basement stairs to our beds, but what if that memory faded away? I could remember the yard, the stubborn Rubik's cube, the kinetic cuckoo clock in the kitchen, the Ford Taurus station wagon, and her orange-colored ash tray filled with extinguished lipstick-stained butts sitting next to her on the table as she sat working through her crossword puzzle with unwavering patience, her crossword dictionary on her right.

I once possessed these kinds of memories for all aspects of my life and had taken them for granted. Robbed of the certainty of their existence, I knew I could never let go of anyone ever again.

The plane departed a couple of days later and, after my arrival in Louisville, Uncle Jim picked me up from the airport and drove to his house, where I would be staying with him.

"She's not doing well," he confided. "They don't think she will make it until Christmas. I don't want you to be surprised when you see her. Visiting hours are over for the day, but we will go first thing tomorrow morning."

We travelled back to his house, making small talk; once we arrived, I dropped my stuff next to the pullout bed he'd made up for me in the living room. We sat up and talked for a bit, me about my job and him about his photography hobby. He was trying to build a portfolio to be able to sell his pictures as stock photos on one of his online photo forums. I could see how much he enjoyed his hobby by the way he spoke about it, clearly hopeful that this new love could become a sustainable career to supplement his retirement. We went to bed somewhat early, since I was tired from my flight, and we knew we had an early morning ahead of us.

The following morning, we headed to the hospital. My inattentiveness and the darkness of the prior evening had allowed me to ignore my surroundings, but when we emerged from the car to head into the hospital, the bitter cold that stung all exposed skin and the surrounding white landscape left no doubt this was Louisville in December.

"The doctors said she is not in any pain," he reminded me as the front automatic doors opened and the warmth of the hospital's heaters met us. "They think she can still hear us even though she isn't responsive."

"We're here to see Alice Ligon," he told the receptionist.

A nearby nurse approached the desk and offered to help.

"I can show them to the room. Which one is she in?"

She chaperoned us down the hall and to Granny's room. Uncle Jim had warned me, and what I saw inside matched his description.

She was on life support, lying lifelessly in the bed, the heart monitor's beep measuring time in the otherwise quiet room. She looked like the grandmother from my memories. This time, though, her stillness did not imply the recharging restfulness of her occasional unintended catnaps in the living room. She wasn't going to wake with a start and laughingly say, "Must have dosed off for a second" to her observers. The machine promised stability, but only at the most basic level.

"Hi, Granny. It's Neil," I whispered, as I stood on the right side of her bed. "I want you to know I'm here."

I held her hand and tried to remember every moment I had spent with her. I remembered bringing up Frescas from the basement to stock the fridge. I remembered her piling my plate with hot pancakes and bacon. I remembered the lunch outings at the nearby Piccadilly. I remembered her showing me how to bait my hook with the squirming minnow on the boat at Rough River.

The beep reminded me I would never hear her voice again. But I still remember.

{chapter 19}

I returned to Atlanta the following day and tried to compartmentalize what I had just seen. The news of Granny's passing reached me a few days later—I winced a goodbye, took a deep breath and put the news aside for later digestion. Work was what was important at that time, so the work routine began again. We were busy, as many lenders sought takers for the money they had allocated to loans in 2005, and their lending standards loosened a bit to accommodate interested borrowers. I used our templates to create Promissory Notes that the lender was issuing. I welcomed the grind, since I once dreaded the end of the day, when my daily efforts for our clients, which I noted on a legal pad, added up to only 5.6 hours. During these busy times, the end result of my electronic tabulation was now 8.5, 9.2, and 10.1 hours, and I left for home in the evenings happy in my newfound security.

I drove back to Aiken a couple of weeks later to enjoy the holidays with my family, and as our busy season at work once again drew to a close, I felt good. My hours were below what was required, but I had been part-time for the first couple of months, so that didn't worry me too much. Chad and Susan were including me socially, Alicia was supplementing this, and even though my ongoing nightmare of train-wreck blind dates was beginning to alarm me, I felt that I could figure out a way to turn things around on that front in the somewhat near future.

When I returned from vacation at the beginning of January, it was time for our performance reviews; one-by-one we were called into the office with Eric and Jay to discuss our review and whether we would receive our merit-based bonus. I knew I wouldn't likely qualify for a bonus, since I had yet to work for a year full time. This meeting would tell me what I needed to focus my efforts on, since I knew my marks would not be exemplary.

We received our assigned times via email and when my appointment arrived, I nervously walked into the office where Jay and Eric sat, reminding myself that the criticism sure to await me was productive criticism and that I should listen carefully and not become defensive.

"We reviewed your file," Eric began. "Your work has definitely improved since you were part-time."

I was already relieved. I felt my latest work was strong, and I was glad they, too, were seeing the improvements.

"But you are still well behind where an attorney of your year should be."

Don't be defensive, I thought. I reminded myself that I needed to keep listening.

"With that in mind, we are going to place you on probation until April."

Panic flooded my brain as I struggled to put my adult self in charge. I had to calm down, show them I was listening and that I was making an effort to integrate their feedback.

"What do I need to do to get off probation?"

"You will have until April to improve your work quality— bring it up to speed with what an attorney of your level should be able to do. We will be carefully monitoring your work from now on to see how you handle your assignments, and if we feel we can see the necessary progress, we will take you off probation. If not, you will need to find another job."

I could tell by looking at them that I was missing something.

"Oh." I collected myself before asking my final question. "Do you think I will be able to improve enough during this time to get off probation?"

Eric's eyes dropped to the floor, and the next words were Jay's.

"You are way behind your class. Right now, what can you actually do?" He paused, though his question was clearly rhetorical.

I think I knew the answer, no matter how desperately I hid from it. I could smile, I could be polite and, as of that week, I could climb the stairs without using the handrails.

"Not everyone is cut out for life at a big firm," he continued. "There are plenty of less challenging legal positions out there that you could be successful in."

The anger boiled inside of me. Of course I was behind my class. I hadn't been working as long as they had. People stopped giving me assignments where I could prove myself months ago. The work I had done recently was good. Maybe if they had given me a chance when I was truly better, I would have been able to show them I could do it now.

I saw the man sitting in front of me and thought he was a smug little prick; a self-righteous man who delivered his damning assessment without an ounce of humanity. I wanted to tell him to go back to his office, with the football trophies from his high school glory days when he was a locally notable five-foot-seven, 160-pound running back or defensive back or whatever, and feel good about himself. If he wanted me to recognize his importance at this institution and make an impassioned plea to save my job, I would never provide him that form of gratification, no matter the stakes. I found him repugnant, and I doubted I was alone.

I didn't see it then as I looked at him in disbelief, my stomach in knots, my face blank with shock, but he was who I was aspiring to be. He was succeeding in a position far superior to my own and I would have to beat unbelievable odds to one day occupy the status that he would soon abandon for bigger successes. He had the large paycheck, the beautiful house and the appropriate familial accessories. I heard at least once a week that his work was terrific and no one who worked with him could deny he was intelligent. He was simply doing his job, eliminating the weak to strengthen the team, and the coldness with which he was expected to deliver corporate justice was a necessary product of his position.

I was shooting the messenger, like I always did. He was right. I didn't know how to do anything. No one had wanted to point it out before because I was friendly, and though I thought that he took too much pleasure in saying what he could have delivered more humanely, at least he was willing to be honest with me, to burst my bubble before I got in serious trouble.

But I was not thankful that day, when I was too dejected to do anything but imagine the physical confrontation that I would have surely lost. Eric finally looked up at the deflated guy in front of him and broke his silence.

"You were so impressive when you were a summer. If you could be that guy again...."

*completely
lost*

{chapter 20}

After they told me who I was not going to be, I wish I could pretend that the days or even months that followed this stomach-punch moment were the finite period of time in which I finally found my road and completed my transformation into the man I was born to be. But the path that I followed did not correspond with my intended schedule, nor did it match the period anyone had medically predicted almost a year and a half before, when I first appeared in an emergency room. Everyone had been wrong.

I was losing my job, the last bit of identity to which I had successfully clung, even during my moments of most horrific failure, and I was trading it for an uncertain and less-promising future. I was tired of others reminding of who I once was when they were not qualified to make such an assessment, but I was far more tired of the present me. My efforts no longer guaranteed success, and the compliments others provided me were framed in the tense of yesterday, with one exception—everyone agreed that I was presently very nice. From what I had seen, this was an entirely useless skill in business and, when coupled with my morose life outlook, it wasn't particularly helpful in my social life, either. The trading of my old identity for this present version, no matter how "nice" it was, was wholly unacceptable, but it was forced upon me with the heartlessness of an older brother trading baseball cards with his younger sibling.

This was temporary, I told myself. I needed to keep buying time until my brain started working again. I'd have to find another job, but once I proved myself, they'd take me back.

I shared the latest revelation with my friends as quickly as I had complained about all of my bad news. I emailed Jill immediately to tell her I had been placed on probation, though it was probation in name only and was intended to allow me time to find another job.

"Oh no! Well, you hate that job anyway," her responding email observed.

"Are you going to stay in law? I wouldn't give up on it. They didn't give you much of a chance there, not even a full year, and I think you could find a job you liked where you could start over."

I felt affirmed in my opinion on this front as I continued to read.

"I have a great legal headhunter you can use if you're interested. She's terrific, and she won't put you in a position where you're going to be miserable to get her finder's fee, like a lot of them will. I trust her completely. I will introduce you to her via email if you want me to."

I told her that I would appreciate that, and she put me in contact with Sandra Keller. Sandra was as friendly as Jill had promised and, knowing Sandra had a responsibility to report potential issues to employers, I carefully omitted why I was looking for another position, emphasizing instead that the big firm had not proven as good a fit as I had hoped. I sent my resume and it was soon making rounds through the Atlanta legal scene.

Despite my concern that news of my accident had reached the legal community beyond my employer, my fears were unfounded, and my resume, with its initial top-tier employer and impressive scholastic achievements from years prior, quickly landed me a couple of interviews at a number of midsized firms. But my interviews began to follow a pattern, beginning with my first one.

The afternoon of my interview, I arrived at the restaurant in the firm's building, nervous and uncertain about what was to occur. A partner, a high level associate and a relatively new associate, all belonging to the team I was hoping to join, came down from their office, we made our introductions and the waiter took us to our table.

After we were seated and put in our drink orders, the partner pulled my resume out, as his coworkers opened their notebooks, and he began. "Looking at your resume, I see you did quite well in school, and I see you are at Irwin Myers now. How do you like it?" the partner questioned.

"I like some of the people I work with, but it is such a large practice that the hours are crazy. The biggest problem is that I still don't feel like I am getting much hands-on experience with anything other than the most basic tasks."

I was trying to learn the skill that almost everyone else had mastered: how to sell oneself in an interview. I had rehearsed my responses in the morning. It played off Irwin Myers' reputation as a sweat shop, which derived mostly from its corporate department's work ethos, though everyone there worked hard and, as such, few outside the firm differentiated its reputation based on the group in question. I fine-tuned my statement to ensure that it did not reflect laziness but instead a concern that I was not achieving professional growth due to a lack of opportunities, demonstrating that I aspired to become a terrific attorney and, in the right circumstances, I would become a model attorney.

Unfortunately, I delivered the message with my eyes turned down at the table, as if I were reading it from a cue card in front of me. I worried they could see my hesitancy and the unending confusion that dwelt in my eyes, so I kept them hidden.

"I am working all of the time, but I do not feel that I'm getting the experience that will be necessary later on," I read.

"That is not surprising," the partner responded. "They have that reputation. I'm going to ask a few questions and try to explain what we do here. I brought along two associates you would be working with, and I think they can explain to you what they do on a daily basis."

The sales pitch began right away. The associates described the office dynamic as friendly and casual, and the partner emphasized that while the starting salary was lower than what I was currently making, there would be many opportunities to gain experience, there would be bonuses to supplement my income, and the billable hours requirement was lower than that of my present position.

"We work hard, but we encourage work-life balance, and our well-rounded associates contribute to our friendly work environment," he explained.

After his cursory explanation of what the position entailed and insight from the associates into what I would be doing, they began to ask me further questions about what I had done while at Irwin Myers. I responded with a description of my role on a few projects where I could, with some effort, make my contributions seem noteworthy. Client confidentiality meant that my vagueness as to which client and what specific project I was referencing was understandable.

Since an attorney of my level was expected to have only a nominal level of knowledge, the interview focused on discovering what kind of growth potential I had. My resume hinted at great promise, and I wanted to avoid dispelling that illusion, though I did have moments where I felt that I could not, in good conscience, maintain the act, usually when I knew I would eventually be uncovered.

"I see you were quite the tennis player in high school," the upper level associate chimed in. "We have quite a few tennis players in the office who play ALTA, though none at your level. Maybe you could hit around with some of them. Have you ever considered playing ALTA?"

ALTA was a wildly popular tennis league in the city that I had avoided completely—just a little more than a year ago, I hadn't measured up particularly well to skilled players confined to a wheel chair. I paled ever so slightly, since I knew any match played with these people of whom he spoke would reveal that I did not possess the skill noted in the "Other" section of my resume, which could call into question the rest of my resume as well. ALTA could reveal me to be a fraud. I quickly began my evasive answer, hiding from the expectations as rapidly as I could.

"Well, I was number two in South Carolina when I was seventeen," I responded. "But that was a long time ago, and I've tried to move on, since that was in the past and I'm not really that guy anymore. I haven't really looked into playing ALTA, but it's something I've heard a lot about."

I felt I had done enough to dispel the myth my resume created, on this front, at least. We continued our friendly lunch, and upon its completion, I shook hands with everyone and headed back to the office. After returning, I further researched the firm with whom I had interviewed. I felt good about the interview, and I anxiously awaited word from Sandra that I had gotten an offer.

A couple days later, she called to inform me that the firm had declined.

"He said you didn't make eye contact through much of the meeting," Sandra told me. "Next time, make sure to make eye contact. He also said that he was puzzled by the fact that you distanced yourself from your tennis accomplishments. That seems to be a strange concern for him to have, but that is how these things go sometimes. Everyone has their personal idiosyncrasies. Don't worry about it; there are a lot of other positions out there, and I've had plenty more interest in your resume, so I'll keep lining up interviews until we find the right fit."

She continued arranging interviews, and I continued bombing them. I mowed down the opportunities offered, whether they were lunches or simple invitations for post-work drinks with employers. Self-confidence was not a talent to list on a resume, so its absence did not serve as a deterrent on paper. But it bled through during face-to-face encounters where they met the real me and guaranteed that all positions lay well outside my reach.

As far as my present job was concerned, my limited skill set was paying dividends. My relative incompetence kept me free of work many days, and my friendly attitude had proven helpful, since I seemed to elicit some emotion akin to sympathy in others, which motivated my employer to provide me with the necessary institutional support for my job search. Eric informed me that it was not imperative for me to be in the office if I had interviews, and when I was, I could spend my time pursuing other job search-related activities like working with legal headhunters.

"We have resources at the firm that you can use in your search. I want you to go speak with Gina, who sits on twenty-four. She's been doing this for a long time, and she understands the legal market and what jobs are available here. Another thing—here is the card for a woman who specializes in people transitioning out of law into other fields. I let her know you would be in contact, so here give her a call."

My firm routine was henceforth completely different than before, with one notable exception. Despite my complete lack of utility to the firm, the prodigious checks continued to be automatically deposited in my checking account. I already felt ashamed about cashing checks that I had never truly deserved over the prior year, and the entitlement that would have eased my concerns never materialized. I tried to convince myself that it was their fault they hadn't provided me with more opportunities to prove myself and that no one had ever confronted me with my failures while I could have fixed them, but Jay's words always reminded me that my failure to learn the necessary skills was the true reason for my predicament. I knew I would forever be indebted to the people who did me the favor of employing me when I was virtually unemployable. I was in the office for seven to eight hours a day, quietly waiting for assignments that rarely came, and I made sure to pursue the career avenues that Eric proposed. I served at the leisure of my kings, and they would tell me how to proceed.

I dutifully spoke with Gina, who, aware of my shortcomings, suggested that I look into a related field, like working as a firm legal librarian. She explained that this was a position for which my law review legal research skills would be helpful, as would my law degree.

I returned to my office and began researching the field online. It seemed to be an adequate way to stay inside the periphery of my big dream job. But to work in this field, it appeared another degree would be necessary, as would job experience, and it was unclear to me how I would get my foot in the door. This path was fraught with uncertainty, but I still looked into where I might need to attend school, though Chad assured me a law degree should be sufficient. I decided this was a worst-case scenario and pursued other avenues with greater vigor.

With the legal librarian position relegated to a worst-case scenario option, I next emailed the woman from Eric's card and explained who I was. Since she was accustomed to handling more established professionals, she passed along my information to one of the women with whom she worked who was better suited for helping someone with less experience. I very soon received an email from the coworker, Wendy Puckett, and we arranged our first meeting.

The day of my appointment, I left my office in the late afternoon and drove to the meeting with Wendy. After I arrived and walked back to Wendy's office, the meeting began with basic small talk. Once I felt comfortable, I presented The Excuse.

"I had a bad car wreck, and I spent the next 3 months in hospitals."

"I'm sorry to hear that. Are you okay?"

"I'm not sure, but I think so. My memory didn't work right at first, but I think it is getting better. I came back to work too soon. Once I kept messing things up, people stopped using me. I think I could do the work now if I had a fresh start, but it's too late."

"I understand. Where are you looking for jobs now?" she asked, trying to transition me out of the past and into the present.

I acquiesced, but not completely. "Well, I am still pursuing legal positions through a headhunter, since I feel pretty certain I could do the work if someone was willing to give me a chance, which I haven't had in a while. But I need to broaden my search, since I have until April to find another job."

"All right, what fields are you interested in?" she asked.

The conversation ground to a screeching halt. I could taste the cake and see the inquisitive faces of rehab again. I had no idea how to answer her question. I was interested in making money and not being fired, but I did not know what field that was.

"I'm, I'm...not real sure," I stammered. "I don't know what other jobs are out there."

She smiled reassuringly. "That is very common for people this early in their careers. There are lots of jobs out there, I promise."

I looked relieved. My problem wasn't unique.

"I'm going to give you this workbook and ask you to complete a couple of exercises in it before our next session," she continued. "Next time, we'll discuss them. Our goal will be determine where your current skills and interests lie, and we can use that as a starting point to determine what areas we should start exploring further. Once we narrow down what kind of jobs interest you, we'll try to find people who work in those fields of interest whom you know and are comfortable talking to. The job search process is going to require some patience, but since you have until April, your goal right now should be to lay the groundwork for your search."

I scheduled our next appointment and left her office optimistic that there were lots of jobs out there, but I was a bit nervous about the term "patience." I knew that I couldn't be patient. If Mom had patiently waited for the hospital in Atlanta to take me, I would still be in rehabilitation. If I had patiently waited for my balance to return completely, I wouldn't be walking. I had overcome problems with force of will—I coped with them by attacking them head on, as rapidly as I could, and watching the fruits of my labor appear before me.

I returned home after my visit with Wendy and, after annihilating another NCAA Football opponent in what I deemed an acceptable and almost necessary break from work, I began my attack on the workbook before me, rapidly answering questions about my interests. One to five scales accompanied the pages of inquiries, five representing the most significance, and though the scale was fractional compared to the pain scale I previously mastered in the hospital, I knew I would soon determine which number corresponded to the magical number seven—the number that would jump-start everything into action.

How important was it that my job was prestigious? Well, it was important, but I knew I would no longer be able to retain employment at a top tier national firm like Irwin Myers, and a "4" seemed to signify some importance while also allowing for my more limited means to acquire a lofty position.

How important was diversity of assignments? I did not hesitate on this question, assigning it a "1" in an attempt to keep it isolated from the other elements. I wanted a straight-forward job, where, through countless repetitions, I could churn out an acceptable work product in my sleep.

I continued on for the next couple of hours, inaccurately documenting my interests to create the perfect template for the job I could achieve. Wendy and I would have lots to talk about next session when she saw the reasonable parameters I created for the job I "wanted." I didn't think it would be that hard. She would be able to direct me to people in that position with whom I could speak and, after hearing of my interest, they would make some inquiries with their company, and I would have a new job.

I was still concerned with the length of time this process would take, and I jumped on every opportunity that crossed my desk. When Chad forwarded me an email he had received from a South Carolina headhunter looking for a transactional lawyer to work in Charleston, I jumped at the chance. I knew this would necessitate taking the South Carolina bar, which was a three-day monster of a test, but I thought that was a problem to worry about later.

I emailed to express my interest, and within a couple of days, I had spoken to the headhunter, who prepared me for a call with a partner in the transactional group with whom I would be working. The partner and I conducted a phone interview, during which I employed all the lessons learned during previous interviews. He didn't hear my downcast eyes and I asked appropriate questions, so they wanted to meet me in person. I flew to Charleston for my interview the next week.

Since Colin was in medical school in Charleston, I planned to spend the weekend there. The schedule had me arriving on Thursday, there was a dinner scheduled for that evening, and then I was to have my interview Friday, after which I planned to spend Friday and Saturday nights at my brother's place before heading back Sunday.

I flew in, grabbed a cab and headed to my hotel, removing my suit from my bag as quickly as possible to prevent wrinkles. In preparation for my dinner plans, I changed into my business casual clothes for the evening, as I had been told to do, and laid out my attire for the next day, making sure my tie matched my suit, and that my socks were the correct color. I requested a wake-up call for the morning, and I set the hotel alarm as well as my cell phone alarm. The office was down the street from the hotel; I reviewed all my materials to make sure I knew exactly where it was so that I would be on time.

That evening, the partner and one of the more senior associates arrived and picked me up at the hotel to take me to dinner. Conversation did not dwell on the firm; instead, we spent the majority of our time discussing how great a city Charleston was. As we ate, the associate pointed out the numerous attractive blondes at the bar.

"That's Charleston for you. We're both married, so we aren't a part of that scene anymore, but a young, single professional guy like you will have a lot of options in this town."

I had no idea what to do with this comment, and I looked around, thinking that this must be a trap. But the waiter came around, and they encouraged me to have another gin and tonic. I figured I would play along, show them I could be one of the guys, and I ordered another drink. By the time dinner concluded, another two empty glasses were in front of me, and I was detailing why one of my girlfriends in law school and I had broken up.

"That's probably enough about that," the associate warned.

"Nonsense," the partner said, laughing. "We're out relaxing."

The next morning's alarm and the accompanying ring of my cell phone alarm had me up, awake, shaved and dressed well in advance of my meeting. The morning headache was not so terrible that I couldn't shake it off, and I arrived in the office waiting room a picture of preparedness: leather folder in hand containing additional copies of my resume and a relaxed look forced onto my face, which, coupled with my well-chosen tie, projected the image of orderly confidence. The receptionist told me they would be with me shortly, and I was soon escorted to my first meeting with the partner from the dinner.

He explained the itinerary, detailing who I would meet with in the firm, and I began my rounds. Everyone was friendly; I met with the attorney with whom I'd had dinner the previous evening, as well as most of the other people who were in the office that day, answering the standard interview questions from people who had prepared for my arrival by scanning my resume the previous evening. After I completed my rounds, I stopped by the partner's office to say goodbye, and he told me they would be in touch.

I strolled around downtown Charleston for a few minutes before heading to my brother's place. The sun was shining, and it was chilly but not particularly cold, despite it being February. I arrived at Colin's place and dropped off my bags, anxious to spend the remainder of the day drinking with him and relaxing.

But I had not released my daydream and moved on to more fun topics even after the second beer, my mind still hard at work playing with a career fantasy. The change of scenery would be perfect, I thought; I could leave the site of my countless failures behind and transition to the more relaxed universe of a mid-sized firm in the more manageable town of Charleston. I thought I could finally succeed here. I sent multiple texts to friends to announce that I had found my next destination even while Colin and I talked about our fantasy football teams. Within an hour, the beer had won.

When I was back in Atlanta a week later, I received an email from the headhunter. The firm had concluded that I was not a good fit, and he wished me all the best in my continued job search. They were apparently not looking for an individual who drank too much at business meetings, talked about his ex-girlfriends, and could not effectively explain what he had done during his previous tenure. I sighed as I flipped through the notebook where I was listing things to remember for future interviews and added excessive drinking to the list of things to avoid.

{chapter 21}

At one point, I believed finding my next job would be easy, but every day proved me wrong. An initial flood of job interviews arranged by Sandra slowed to a trickle, and my days became less and less productive. I waited in anticipation for Sandra to send another interview my way, and I looked through my notes regarding past interview failures. Make eye contact. Ask more questions about their company. Don't get drunk. My daily existence was a training exercise for my next interview.

On occasion, the office was busy enough that an assignment came across my desk that required my help. Beyond those rare occurrences, I sporadically searched for jobs online, went to lunch with Chad and Susan whenever they could make time, and spent the rest of my day discovering my strengths and interests with the help of Wendy's books. How important is monetary compensation? Even after the rash of failed interviews, I could definitely still find a job where the pay provided an incentive that qualified as a "4."

Unfortunately for me, Chad and Susan frequently stayed busy, limiting our lunch opportunities to once a week at most, and I could only spend so much time each day pretending that I was okay making less money at a less prestigious job. Thus, I sat in my office with the door closed with copious amounts of free time, useless to my employer and undesired by others, feeling that my presence was an inconvenience for everyone. I spent some of my downtime searching iTunes for The Arctic Monkeys' latest CD or assorted rap songs that I could download to my iPod. But that only took a few minutes, and time dragged as I sat in my solitary confinement and hoped to God Sandra could find another job for which I could interview.

I needed to keep myself busy to avoid continuing my day-long worries about potential problems finding future employment. I had Sandra helping me with that, and I was working with Wendy to find other avenues to explore, so I didn't see what else I could do on that front. My employer didn't need or want my help with anything, since no one trusted my work, and I was forced to search for meaning elsewhere.

Robbed of a job to worry about, I applied my neurosis liberally to my life outside of the office. The absence of a girlfriend continued to torment me; I had been single since Amy left and was uncomfortable spending significant time alone with my thoughts. Additionally, though my social group had expanded to include Jill and, by extension, all of her friends, I still had very few people in the Atlanta area who considered me a friend. With seemingly no other options, I set about spending my free time at the office trying to determine the best way to remedy these problems.

The dating issue had stubbornly refused to resolve itself during the months preceding my probation. People set me up on blind dates, but the women who showed up moved from enthusiasm about their friend's selection to horror, as I poured out bloodcurdling details of my wreck injuries and moaned about the new problems I now faced. My friends encouraged me to limit my exploration of these topics, since tales of surgery were not an aphrodisiac.

After numerous failed efforts, I took their advice to heart and approached my next date, arranged with Alicia Stone's help, with a verbal tentativeness I hoped would keep me from instantly revealing all of my issues. My initial email exchange with this woman worried me a bit; my desire to lower expectations far enough that I might actually exceed them meant the emails were peppered with references to my unimpressive physical appearance, and she had become quite alarmed that I might not be up to her standards.

I answered her concerns with the precision of a politician, resorting to my fallback position. "I was once known as the hot TA, so I don't think I'm bad to look at."

Known by whom? And I was once a lot of things that I had proven, to a near certainty, I would never be again. My claim was pathetic, but it echoed my life strategy. I was insistent on pretending to be the person I had only heard about, and since I still looked the same, I focused on this. The opinion that might have been voiced by 22-year-old women two years before took on a significance that they could never have imagined. Had they in fact made such a statement? It didn't matter anymore.

We weren't off to a promising start, but I chalked it up to early jitters, and we arranged to meet at the Cheesecake Factory, which was right up the road from me. When she walked in, I recognized her from the picture she had sent me. The waiter led us to our seats, and we began to talk.

"Alicia and I were talking at a house party I was at," she explained. "When she found out I was from Atlanta, she said she had a really cool guy friend who lived here and she asked me for my number and email address so that she could give it to you. I figured, what the hell, why not?"

"I'm glad you did," I told her, hoping I was effectively hiding my nervousness.

The waiter came around and took our orders. She ordered one of the salads, while I settled on the Louisiana Chicken Pasta. The food came out quickly and we ate as we continued to talk. I was a lawyer. I hoped she was impressed, though she showed no indication, and I quickly steered the conversation back to her.

"So I went to this other house party with a guy friend," her story began. "And we were having fun and all. Then I was standing on the porch talking with some people when a girl came outside, all pissed. She was his ex-girlfriend, apparently. And she was mad as hell."

I looked down at my plate. This wasn't going well. Just keep quiet, I thought.

"Then all of a sudden she was up in my face screaming at me," she continued.

"Well, it happens," I responded.

"She was like, 'You were the bitch he was cheating with, weren't you?'"

I was horrified but kept still, as if the ferocious tale unfolding in front of me might forget about me and stop charging ahead.

"And I was like, 'I don't know what you're talking about. Get out of my face.'"

"Well, it happens," I interjected, still entirely at a loss for words.

"And then she came after me and we started fighting on the porch until a couple of the guys came out and broke it up."

"Well, it happens."

"And so my shirt was all torn and I was still screaming at her as the guys pulled us apart."

"Well, it happens."

She paused from her Jerry Springer story, and lifted the fork with speared greens to her mouth, cleared its tines between her front teeth, chewed twice and swallowed. I hoped that the story was mercifully over. I was trying to decide how to change the subject, when I realized she wasn't quite done. With the fork in her right hand, she rotated it to face me and placed her thumb behind the business end of the implement.

"If you say 'it happens' one more time, I'll stab you in the eye with this fork."

Dinner ended without homicide, and I emailed her the following day to see if she would be interested in a second date, which she declined through her silence. I had become the guy so desperate for companionship that I was willing to risk not only the disdain of my date, but my physical wellbeing as well. From that point on, I knew that until I could straighten out other parts of my life, my dating life needed to take a back seat to everything else.

Unfortunately, there were not a lot of avenues remaining. My professional life was stalling; I could not accelerate my healing; and my pursuit of happiness was not to include women, at least not in the near future. I did, however, have significant amounts of free time that I still needed to fill.

I decided that it was time to find more people I could hang out with, and at Chad's suggestion, I looked into the UVa Club of Atlanta, the University's local alumni group. I found their website and looked for sports offerings. I was specifically interested in basketball, since I remained above average height, which I thought would offset balance and coordination issues, and I might be useful to the team so long as I was willing to run the floor, set picks, and grab rebounds. Unthinkingly, I was running toward the social crutch I had once propped myself up with, outlets for my athleticism, even when aptitudes in this area no longer remained.

The site mentioned that anyone with an interest in intramurals should contact Jamie Barlow, who was in charge of club intramural teams, so during the midst of my daily tedium, I became involved with the University alumni group. I composed my email, avoiding my standard tactic of overwhelming the recipient with stories about my wreck. I thought maybe this venue would be an opportunity to create a new identity, one that didn't dwell on the past.

"Hi. My name is Neil Ligon, class of 2001. Haven't joined the alumni group yet but plan to in the next couple of days. I am finally slow at work, am somewhat new to the area, and decided to actually start trying to integrate myself into the community. I was wondering what teams you all have and if any of those teams are in need of participants. Oh, and I was wondering if you have a basketball team. I am no longer athletic, but I like to pretend. Thanks."

Jamie responded that day with a friendly, inclusive email that I would come to know as her trademark, despite her protestations throughout the following seasons claiming she wasn't really all that nice.

"Glad to hear you're interested in joining up! Currently we're doing bowling on Tuesday nights and volleyball on Thursday nights, and then in the spring we'll be doing softball on Thursday nights, kickball on Saturdays and potentially flag football on Mondays. Any of these interest you?"

I was a terrible bowler, but I had played volleyball on the sand courts behind my dorm my freshman year of college, so I expressed interest in the spring sports, and I joined the volleyball team but warned her that I would not be particularly good.

"If it helps, we have yet to actually win a game this season, so there's little pressure to be good," she assured me.

The gym was in an area of Atlanta I was unfamiliar with, but I still managed to find it by our assigned time. During warm-ups, I introduced myself to my teammates, who were all friendly upon my introduction, and we discussed when we graduated, our jobs and other such standard topics, all while I tried to relearn how to bump the volleyball in the intended direction.

As the game began, even with the lack of pressure, I was horrible. My vertical, which was never my strength thanks to banjo-string-tight hamstrings and terrible tennis knees, was now a victim of my unwillingness to commit fully to jumping—I was still terrified of falling over due to suspect balance. Though my fingertips reached the top of the tape at the net when I stood flat-footed, I could barely get my hands all the way over the net when I jumped, making my attempts to spike the ball sail long and all attempts to block a shot comically ineffective.

I became frustrated at times with my ineptitude, but when I was focused on the moment, on the camaraderie fueled by a group striving toward a common goal, I had fun. Compliments were liberally distributed among our team, and a serve that came off the side of my hand and dropped in for an ace garnered supportive fanfare, while my serve into the net that followed did not elicit the disgust from others that it did from me. The stronger players on the team kept us competitive but were not enough to save us, and we lost both games. As we headed for the exits at the gym, I thanked Jamie for inviting me to play and apologized for being so terrible.

"It was helpful to have another tall guy, and you played fine," she assured me. "Thanks for coming out. You should join us for the season. The games are most Wednesdays at this gym; I'll send you the schedule. We're getting better, and I think we're going to win at least once this season. I'll let you know about the other teams and when we start our spring season, too."

This seemed promising. It was an opportunity to use my athletic drive but didn't punish me for the fact that athleticism no longer accompanied my desire to compete. Even though I had been a complete detriment to the team, no one made a big deal about it and I enjoyed myself throughout the match. It was somehow surprising to me that no one made fun of how terrible I was, even though no one had explicitly derided my efforts in the other areas of my life,. My ego was as fragile as my face.

Everyone at volleyball was close to my age, and we all had at least one thing in common: an apparent tie to Mr. Jefferson's university. This was something to look forward to. Maybe something as simple as intramural sports was the escape I had been missing.

{chapter 22}

Every day I reminded myself of the need for patience. Despite my disdain for passively waiting, I knew my life wouldn't magically come together in a few months. From my days of rehab and intermittent web research on head injury, I knew I would continue healing measurably for the next five years, and even then, the healing would continue for the rest of my life, though rarely in noticeable increments. Every new day's arrival meant I was stronger than before—surviving was healing.

Feeling limited by my apartment gym, I had joined a nearby Crunch Fitness to expand my efforts and was working out there with my trainer, at 6:00 in the morning, for one hour twice a week to add muscle stamina, strengthen my struggling left side, and further develop core body strength to help my balance. I supplemented these sessions with my own workouts at the gym anywhere from one to three times a week. I was creating a social life incrementally, supplementing my friendships with Chad and Susan with Alicia's friends and Jill's friends. I now had UVaClub volleyball to occupy me, and softball and kickball were soon to follow. I had resumes circulating through Sandra. I met with Wendy to refine my job search outside the legal field. My daily routine at work was a model of efficiency, despite the fact that my well-compensated efforts were rarely of any use to anyone besides me.

Nonetheless, this self-absorbed life detour, still in its earliest stages, did not provide an adequate number of distractions, and an unending quest for self-betterment left moments in every day when I was too tired to continue toward a goal that never seemed to draw closer. My Hotmail account became my tour guide during those moments, providing numerous opportunities to escape my universe. I emailed friends and planned visits with those who wrote me back. I was a virtual voyeur into all my friend's lives until they would invite me in and let me see their world in person. I looked everywhere else but wouldn't open my eyes to what lay in front of me until I ran out of excuses to look away.

After a brief trip to visit a friend out West, I returned to Atlanta, with two somewhat promising job prospects; unfortunately, the efficiency with which I had run through my previous opportunities hinted that these two might be the only remaining firms in the city with whom I might have a chance. I had completed multiple interviews with both and could tell that I was near the last round of interviews, leaving me ever hopeful that I would finally make the last cut and slide into a job. My resume was eye-catching and, with the help my interviewing notebook, I was avoiding my classic interview mistakes. I felt like a big break was right around the corner.

The firm for whom I most wanted to work scheduled a lunch meeting at a nearby Outback, where I was to meet with the partner I would work under and one of the firm's associates. I made it to the restaurant a couple of minutes before they did and fidgeted nervously while I awaited their arrival. The partner made it first.

"Hi, Neil. It's good to see you. Let's grab a table." As we sat down at our table, he explained that some things had come up. "Adam got tied up on a conference call, so he will be running a little bit late. Let's go ahead and order, and he'll join us a little bit later."

The waiter came to take our drink order and, remembering my notebook, I stuck with a Coke. It was also twelve-thirty in the afternoon.

The conversation began smoothly, and he casually probed my understanding of real estate law. I answered every question as succinctly as possible. After a few minutes of relaxed questions, while he was discussing lending work, he slipped in the first tough question.

"Why do banks use land as collateral for their loans? You just finished telling me that you have worked on loan modifications so that the borrower will not default, since the banks do not want to own land. So why would they use land as the collateral, then? What is the bank truly worried about?"

He finished, and I knew that this job rode on my answer. I left the question out there lingering for about fifteen seconds, breaking the silence intermittently with "um" and "well," promising additional information that never followed. I wracked my brain for every piece of information I could pull from my time at Irwin Myers, and I remembered the Assignment of Rents documents they usually had me create using the lender's form document. I blurted it out as the best guess I had.

"I think they are concerned with the income stream the property generates, not the property itself," I finally answered.

"Yes!" He seemed genuinely happy that I had answered correctly. "That's right. I'm impressed you knew that. So many young attorneys forget that is what actually matters."

I knew I had aced the interview. Absent some sort of tragic misstep on my part, I had the job in hand. The conversation continued on at a leisurely pace, and I felt myself begin to relax. He discussed his background a bit and talked about the firm, but it was an easygoing conversation without further potential pitfalls.

After he shared some personal stories from the beginning of his time as an attorney, he casually asked, "Is there anything about you that you think I should know?"

"Well, you have my resume and I think that explains my educational background," I answered, confused as to what he meant. "If you have any questions in particular, please let me know, and I will clarify anything that has caused confusion."

"No, I think I understand your resume, and we've discussed your time at Irwin Myers in depth. I wanted to give you a chance to tell me anything you feel is important that is not on the resume."

I thought for a moment that he must have known about the wreck. This must be a test. Why else would he ask such a thinly veiled question?

Before I confessed, I reminded myself that I always thought people knew about my wreck. What haunted me was invisible to everyone else. Mom had emphasized that unless I told people, they would not know. It was me projecting onto him, and I told myself that he couldn't tell.

Since I thought it was all in my head, after a slight hesitation, I answered carefully, "Um, not that I can think of."

The uncomfortable pause that followed lasted only a few seconds before Adam walked through the door and headed for our table. He quickly introduced himself and apologized for being late.

"I could not get off that conference call. I am terribly sorry. Can we extend this a few minutes? Maybe we can grab coffee or dessert?"

I agreed to lengthen the meeting, since I believed I was drawing closer to leaving with that elusive offer in hand. After we put in our dessert order, I discussed the office dynamics with Adam. With dessert sitting in front of us, and my conversation with him winding down, the partner once again addressed me.

"I've enjoyed talking with you today, Neil. We would like you to schedule a meeting with an industrial psychologist we use in the next week or so, if that's possible."

Warning bells immediately went off in my head. Adam's sudden appearance had distracted me, but it was clear that the partner did know about my wreck. What had they heard about me that they wanted me to meet with this person? Maybe they had heard about everything. The partner noticed my panic and quickly tried to calm me down.

"We do this with all of our attorneys. We want to know what kind of learning style you have and how you react to criticism to make sure you'll fit in well with the rest of the office, and we want to know how to best provide you feedback should you join our firm."

I was not convinced. This sounded like a trap. I feared this test would somehow reveal that my memory still did not work right. But maybe it did work now. I couldn't even tell anymore.

"Adam took it, didn't you?" the partner said to his colleague.

"It's been a while, but I remember taking it before I started. It wasn't bad. It took a couple of hours, but it really wasn't a big deal."

Lunch concluded, and the partner handed me his card.

"Call my secretary and get the number for the psychologist. Once you get the number from her, give him a call and schedule your appointment as soon as you can. I'm sorry that lunch went over our scheduled time, but as you know, that is the way things go with clients sometimes."

I slid into my car, on edge and confused, and returned to my office. The partner had commented on my perceptive answer to his question, which had to be a good sign. But I didn't understand why I needed to take a personality test. I tried to explain the request away. Adam had taken it, so it had to be one of those quirky things people in this particular small office had to go through.

Still, I was already tired of all of the tests. Everything, no matter how simple, was a test. Could I climb the stairs while not looking down at my feet? Could I jump without falling over? Could I remember the lyrics to the song I'd heard on my car ride in to work? Could I run the 5K in under thirty minutes? I was worn out from my own tests, and potential employers', once content to simply test me in interviews, where I could fail in the moment and then move on, were now formalizing the process so that they could create a more permanent written record of my inadequacies.

Once I got back to the office that afternoon, I was still tense from lunch, but I was desperate to conclude the process and either receive a rejection or an offer, so I called his secretary for the psychologist's number. After speaking with the psychologist's receptionist, the test was scheduled for the following Tuesday. I was too nervous about the test to consider the possibility that I was moving closer to a job offer.

The morning of the test, I left my apartment and traveled to the building about a mile up the street from me. The first part of the exam was the Wonderlic Personnel Test, the intelligence test usually given to NFL players at the combine—fifty questions in twelve minutes. I answered forty-one of them and hoped this would be enough. The next portion, as promised, tested my learning style. I systematically went through the questions and, following the test instructions, assessed which of the choices best described my response to whatever the particular question asked.

The questions were supposed to show everyone my personality, and I wanted to convey a hard-working, self-confident person who demonstrated leadership abilities but was also a terrific team player, since this was clearly who they hoped to hire. Still, the psychologist had warned me to be honest, or my answers would not be consistent and the test would be of no use to them. I wanted the results to guarantee that they would hire me, but I also knew that skewed test results would almost certainly take me out of contention for the position.

This time, I did not rush my answers. I analyzed each question carefully, and I answered honestly, except when I thought an honest answer would specifically show me to be lazy. After I completed the exam, I spoke with the psychologist for a few minutes.

"I will send your results along, but I don't see anything that would worry them," he told me.

I was relieved. I had been extraordinarily nervous in the days leading up to the exam. If there was a test out there that could accurately measure whether you could do your job, I wasn't sure I could pass it, and this had sounded like such a test. But I was healed enough that the test showed I was okay.

Since I still wasn't sure I'd earned the position, I continued with my follow-up interviews for the second firm, Cole Hyde. They scheduled my interviews for the following week and, after I parked, I walked up to the modest four-story building that housed the firm, situated less than a mile up the street from my apartment. It was a fairly small office of about thirty-five attorneys and another fifteen or so support staff. The attorneys were divided fairly evenly between the litigation practice, which focused primarily on family law, and the transactional practice, which was concerned mostly with development work.

I met with Alan, the founding partner in the transactional department, first, before touring the office. Though not particularly big in stature, he filled space. He left his chair and strode with purpose to greet me at his door.

"Come in," he boomed in what sounded to me like a Northeastern accent of some sort as he shut the door behind me. "I'll let you know what we're looking for, and then you'll meet some of the other people you would work with."

I took a seat in front of him, on the other side of his desk, trying not to squirm as I became the momentary object of his focused intensity, and he began to discuss the job.

"You'll be primarily working with me, but you'll also help out the other partners when they need you. We definitely have the work to keep you busy." He paused, but only briefly. "I handle a lot of time-share development work, and I'm looking for someone to work with me and become familiar with the work so they can take the lead on some of these developments. This is a huge industry, and we are a leader in the field. I speak at industry conferences all the time; in fact, I am speaking at one in Hilton Head in a couple of weeks. I'm looking for someone to work with me and learn the ropes so they can eventually take over this practice. Have you done any development work before?"

"Not much," I confessed. "But it looks really interesting. One of the frustrating things about the lending practice I'm currently in is that our clients refinance so rapidly, the documents I am creating are rarely ever in force even a few months after I work on them. I think it would be nice to be able to physically see what my work made possible."

"Exactly," he responded. "It's a fast-paced practice, but I will work with you and let you sit in on conference calls with clients and really get to know the clients we work with."

This was a perfect time to interject one of my stock answers.

"Great. That is one of the things I feel like I'm really missing out on. I don't get much client contact. All I'm doing is modifying template documents."

"I can promise you, that will not be a problem around here. This firm is growing fast, and we may be expanding into other markets soon. We need more good attorneys to handle all of our new work. I see you were on law review, too, so I know you can write and won't have a problem doing the work."

I wasn't as sure, but I nodded in agreement anyway.

"Everything around here is top of the line. We have this new system where you can log in to your profile from home and pull up your email. We have world-class technical support around here," he raved.

I did my best to hide my lack of amazement at this technology. I had seen the other world, and my expectations did not align with my abilities. Even as that world cast me out, I still remembered the good from our time together, and this colored my perception of my suitors. At my current job, we always had the "new" log-in system that he was now touting, and I had twenty-four hour a day computer support on speed dial.

Still, this wasn't bad. Maybe I was getting in on the ground floor of a firm that would soon become one of the giants in the legal market in Atlanta. I could work hard and become the heir to this seemingly lucrative practice.

He continued, interrupting my grandiose visions of the future, "I'm going to need you to take the South Carolina bar, because we do a lot of work in South Carolina. If you don't pass it, it isn't a big deal, but I will want you to take it. Now, we can't pay you like the big firms do, but we do not require the same hours."

"What is the billable hour requirement?" I asked as he opened the door to take me to the next person's office.

"It is a two thousand billable hour requirement, and, with the work we have, you won't have any problems reaching that number."

This was no different than Irwin Myers hour requirement, despite the lower salary, and that made me nervous. But he quickly did his best to assuage my concerns on this front.

"If you miss two thousand, it is no big deal."

One of the associates was walking by, and he quickly grabbed his attention. "Jerry, what time do you leave by?"

"I get in later, so I am usually here until around six, but I am always gone by seven," came Jerry's response.

"I bet no one around your firm can say that," the partner said to me as he walked me to the next interview.

"After you finish the interviews, I will have you talk with Joyce, who handles office administration. She can explain our medical benefits plan, which provides the best coverage, and answer any questions about that, and then we can talk."

After speaking with five of the individuals who were members of the transactional team, I concluded my interview tour of the office and went in to speak with Joyce, who discussed the firm's PPO and dental health plans before she walked me back to Alan's office.

I thought the interviews had gone well, and when he saw that I looked pleased, he wasted no time.

"I am serious about hiring someone, and I want to be sure you're interested in working here, too. I need to talk with the people you met with today to make sure they are comfortable with you. But, if we were to make an offer, would you accept?"

I was a bit taken aback. I liked the people I had met, and my headhunter assured me she had not heard anything negative about the firm, but I did not have any of the details about the offer, including the starting salary, and I tried to backpedal as rapidly as possible without seeming disinterested.

"Everyone I met with today seemed like they would be good to work with, and I am definitely interested in a position here. I think I mentioned this before, but I need to give my employer two weeks' notice, and I am in a friend's wedding at the end of April. What would the offered starting salary be?" I asked, hoping something in my question would buy me some time.

He rapidly okayed my time restrictions and spit out a narrow dollar range for the salary, foiling my strategy.

I kept hoping he would notice my discomfort and let me off the hook, but I was not so fortunate. He had made me a non-offer offer. I had no idea how I was supposed to respond. Though I was excited that I possibly had two firms who wanted me, I simply wanted to dwell on that fact for a few days before making a decision one way or another, and committing to take a position which had not even been officially offered felt inappropriate.

Still, though the starting salary was lower than I had hoped, maybe this was the best I could do, and I did not want to lose all of my prospects and be stuck unemployed. I thought I had done well in my interview at the other firm, and I had not heard back from them about their slightly better compensated position. I didn't want to commit myself to a lower offer unless I was out of options, but I also didn't want to alienate the man who was giving me the closest thing to an offer I had received.

I tried to talk myself into it, even as I remained entirely confused about how to respond. The work at this firm seemed pretty steady, and he had assured me that I would work fewer hours, so maybe this was the perfect place to rejuvenate my career. And maybe the other firm had already decided not to make me an offer. What would I do if I lost both opportunities? I had to be out of opportunities with as many interviews as I had blown. I needed some time to figure out what my actual options were.

"I need to think about it," I finally answered, trying to hide my uncertainty. "I like the idea of doing development work, and I'm excited about the possibility of working closely with someone like you who is an expert in the field. I don't mean to sound wishy-washy, but I need to really think about it carefully before I make such a big decision."

"That's fine. I will talk to the people you interviewed with, and then I will get back to you. If we make you an offer, I will need an answer, since we are interviewing quite a few candidates for our open positions."

He held out his hand, and I shook it and thanked him before, careful not appear as if I were running, I moved rapidly toward the lobby and the safety of the accompanying elevator. As the elevator descended one floor to ground level, I took a deep breath. After two and a half months of interviews, I almost had my first offer. Granted, this wasn't the job I wanted, but it was definitely better than nothing and I could use it as a jumping-off point for my still fledgling career.

{chapter 23}

With the end of my probation period fast approaching, my work conundrum had been making me especially jumpy. I knew I had Kevin's wedding to look forward to very soon and, during the day, I reviewed my potential trip itinerary and the emails from all my friends. At night, though, I struggled to sleep, as nightmarish visions of an unemployed future ran through my head. I had saved no money for my present uses and, though I had maxed out my 401K, I was for all practical purposes broke.

Initially, I wondered how this could be. Sure, I ate out all of the time, my student loans ran me almost $500 a month, my car payment was $540 a month and I was saving a ton of money for my 401K, but I still didn't understand how I ran through the large bi-monthly paycheck so rapidly. I tossed and turned in my bed at night, envisioning my universe without a paycheck. I wouldn't be able to live.

I knew that upon my grandmother's passing, my father's share of the inheritance had been split between me and my brother, and it had been far more sizable than I thought possible, enough to pay off my private student loans and for a substantial down payment on a house. But her estate was still being settled, and this money would remain unavailable to me for the near future, and it felt like blood money anyway. It was simply another example of me profiting from my father's death, much like the life insurance and social security payments Mom used to maintain our childhood lifestyle in such a manner that nothing was missing, except for him.

In those days, guilt faded rapidly with the purchase of every shiny new object I asked for and received, beginning with the car I eventually parked at the bottom of the interstate. Maybe it was karma that fueled that car and my future's destruction that day, since I'd never deserved any of the things that had been so freely given to me. And yet, here I was again, soon to be dependent on support I shouldn't have received.

I was trading in a palatable guilt for one that I could not stomach. I knew I'd never deserved my paycheck, but I quieted the doubt by reminding myself how much money my employer was making. They weren't missing the paychecks they tossed my way. But faced with a jobless future, I would have to live on a bridge loan from Mom, a public school teacher, until the monetary reward for my father's and grandmother's deaths arrived, and that would merely delay my move onto the familial dole. During those nights, my eyes screwed shut, my pulse racing, I knew I was millimeters away from permanently becoming the burden I had temporarily been in the hospital.

My nightly journey down this self-loathing path was mercifully cut short. A few days after my interview at the second firm, my phone rang with good news. They extended me an offer and asked for an answer by the end of the week. I finally had the proverbial bird in the hand, but even with the relief it brought, I still preferred the other position.

"I haven't heard back from them yet," Sandra informed me when I called her with the news of my offer and asked about the other firm. "I will try to get an answer as soon as I can."

The week wore on, and I spent my time in the office reading through the emails flying about for Kevin's wedding, buying iTunes songs, and incessantly fidgeting. With my deadline almost upon me, I tried to extend the time period previously discussed by a few extra days.

"I know I told you that I would have my answer by the end of this week, but is there any way I could get an extension?" I emailed Alan. "This will be a huge move, and I want to be absolutely sure that I am comfortable with everything before I make this jump."

The email bought me until midweek the next week, and I called to tell Sandra to let the firm know I needed an answer by Monday of the next week. When she informed them of my deadline, they said they would let her know by then. They delivered their answer to her the next day, and she called to tell me.

"They have decided to pass. The people you met with really liked you and thought you would be a good fit, but they didn't feel as if you had enough experience. I know, I have no idea why they would interview you if they needed a fourth year attorney, but, apparently, that is what they concluded they need. The partner also said that they knew about a bad wreck you were in, and it worried them that you hadn't been forthright about that. Oh well, it doesn't matter now. You can take that other position and not have to worry about having to make a tough decision."

My wreck was not a secret to anyone who looked deep enough. Maybe I had bombed the test I had taken for them. Maybe the rehabilitation magazine cover had shown up in a Google search. Maybe someone had heard the story while I still proudly told it over beers or in our break room and had alerted them to the potential problem. I would never know.

Regardless, my future had been decided. I was to re-launch my professional identity from the platform I had been given. It seemed I would finally have an opportunity to learn what I was doing at the other firm. I forced myself to look okay with the turn of events as I tried to imagine my re-emergence from employment purgatory back onto the big stage, where everyone would marvel at my physical recovery as well as my career renaissance.

With that, I picked up the phone and called my new employer.

"Cole Hyde," a cheerful voice informed me.

"Hi, this is Neil Ligon. May I speak with Alan, please?"

"One moment, please," the receptionist answered me.

The phone rang twice before he answered it.

"Neil, this is Alan. What can I do for you?"

"Mr. Cole, I appreciate your willingness to extend my decision deadline, and I am happy to tell you that, after careful thought, I have decided to accept your offer. I look forward to the opportunity to work with you."

I worried that perhaps he had decided to revoke the offer. I had nothing in writing. I had no legal recourse if he did. I waited anxiously for his response.

"Glad to hear it. I will have Joyce email you all the paperwork, and you need to sign everything and send it back to us. I have a client call here in a few minutes, so I have to go, but I am glad you will be joining us."

The line went dead after our goodbyes. This was the first full-time job offer I could ever remember receiving, and yet there was no sense of accomplishment to accompany the call's termination. The pride I must have felt when offers for summer internships poured in after my interviews in law school was not mine that day.

Was it the embarrassment that I had begun a professional regression of sorts? An inability to follow the path my past had set in front of me? That's what it felt like at first. But with the wisdom of hindsight, another issue was identifiable.

The final two employment candidates had both analyzed me, and only the second one, relying on my resume and a blind belief that I was the law review talent I probably wasn't anymore, accepted me. The first one had been more diligent with their research, and so they knew me better and rejected me. Finding a job at a Buckhead law firm known throughout the city for their expertise in development work was still an impressive accomplishment for most lawyers. But once again, it wasn't mine. I had obtained this job because of my resume, because of who I had once been.

{chapter 24}

With my acceptance official, I emailed Chad and Susan to let them know my news, and I walked down to Eric's office, resignation in hand. It was time to officially end my farcical existence at Irwin Myers. I timidly knocked before peeking around the corner of the door frame.

"Come in, Neil. What can I do for you?"

"Eric, I wanted to provide you with my two week notice of my resignation." For the first time, my eyes met his unflinchingly as I passed the piece of paper to him across his large desk. I was ending my days of being a burden to him.

"My last day will be March 17. I have taken a position with Cole Hyde."

"Congratulations to you!" he boomed. It was easy to see that he was happy for me. I knew he, too, was aware that my probationary period was coming to a close, and my announcement saved him from the unpleasantness of having to fire me.

"They have an excellent reputation for their work with timeshare developers. I think this will be a great opportunity for you."

I carefully gathered my thoughts before I spoke. I owed him so much for keeping my job open while I was in the hospital, for keeping me on at the firm even as I struggled and for giving me these months to find another position. I wanted to deliver a genuine thank you that accurately conveyed my gratitude while avoiding false flattery. Even with the extra time I took, my next statement sounded like a rejected greeting card.

"I really, really appreciate everything you have done for me. I know you did things for me that you didn't have to do, and I will always be thankful for my time here and all of the opportunities I had while I worked here. I'm sorry that I couldn't live up to expectations, and I know I am the only one responsible for that. I will truly miss everyone I had the chance to work with, and I wish you the best of luck in the future."

He looked back at me while I delivered my goodbye monologue, and as I finally finished, he delivered his response in as kindly a manner as possible, at his customary volume. It was as if he hoped his words could be a salve for the sting of the inescapable reality I was standing before him briefly accepting.

"I'm sorry this didn't work out, Neil. I think you will make an excellent attorney, and it's unfortunate that you will not be continuing on with us. I've been involved in my firm's summer intern program for twenty-five years, and you were the best summer associate I ever saw." An uncomfortable pause followed before he resumed with the business portion of our discussion.

"I will forward this on to Gina in HR, and she will be in contact with you to schedule an exit interview and let you know anything else she needs from you. Best of luck to you in your new job, and please stay in touch."

After months of worrying and wondering if I would be there tomorrow, I finally knew precisely when it would end. I returned to my desk, and waited for the relief to arrive. It was finally over. I had lived so much of my free time in Atlanta scared of my friends' introductions, unsure of how to deal with the inevitable.

"What do you do?" the friendly new face always asked.

"I'm an attorney," I would respond.

"Oh, where do you work?" came the inevitable next question.

"Irwin Myers."

And before I could correct the misconception my answer created, I was neck deep in a lie. I could not remedy the confusion that my answer caused without a detailed description of my incompetence and the intervening cause that had caused my intelligence to fade.

"Oh, that is a very good firm. What area do you practice in?"

"I work for the real estate department, but I'm so junior I really don't know how to do much."

"Stop being modest! That is a very impressive place."

With that, we then moved on to subjects of greater import, like their careers or how we both came to know our mutual friend, and in my mind, the misunderstanding became the cornerstone of any future interaction.

This conversation was scripted for me, and I read my lines almost once a week. Initially, I fought it—I explained to my newest acquaintance the problems with my answer. I found pitying eyes, uncomfortable squirming and, on occasion, a need to excuse himself or herself to say hello to a newly discovered friend across the room. With social coaching from Mom and other friends, I did my best to abandon unnecessary detail, answering succinctly with my company name and my title and, in my new script, one sentence of explanation took the place of a chapter of clarification.

Surely, I would now welcome the chance to simply give my firm's name without feeling the burn of an inextinguishable guilt over the confusion I was causing. I had spent the last year of my life petrified at the thought of being fired. With this great weight lifted, I could finally experience freedom from expectations I could never meet and calm down and enjoy things.

Still, the relief didn't come when I sank down into my chair. Two problems remained. The first one that haunted me was whether I could be successful in my new job. I hadn't really been learning much at Irwin Myers, and Alan might expect knowledge I didn't have. I also couldn't remember much of what I learned in law school, even if what I learned there could have helped me, which I suspected was not the case.

Nevertheless, I finally had a fresh start, and the work I would be doing at Cole Hyde was not the same as what I claimed to do at Irwin Myers. This would give me some time to catch up before the expectations regarding what I could do rose too high. I thought this would probably be enough.

The second issue wasn't as easily dispatched. My job defined me. No matter how much I openly loathed it and hated the fact that every day it reminded me of all my inadequacies, I enjoyed the rubber stamp seal of approval that my employer's name provided. Did the guilt wrack me even as I mentioned it? Yes, it did. But without that business card, what was left to admire? There wasn't even anything left to respect. My athleticism was barely present. I couldn't get a second look from a woman to save my life, and, as of March 17, I would no longer have an impressive job and the superfluous money that accompanied it. What else mattered?

Chad's knock on my door ended my introspection. It opened, and he moved into the office and half-shut the door. "Congratulations on the new job. Celebratory lunch with me and Susan next Wednesday? I was thinking maybe we could try this new place in the Highlands I've been hearing about."

"Sure, sounds good to me. Looking forward to it," I answered.

"It sounds like you'll be working right down the street from where you live at your new job, which I'm sure will be nice," he added. "I'm sick of my commute. Almost every morning, there is a wreck that backs everything up."

Our previous discussions regarding the position, at the time I was interviewing, meant that no further analysis of the job was necessary, since I had already shared everything I knew. He was being a friend, pretending that this was on my terms, highlighting the positive while I sat overwhelmed by the negative. I wasn't jealous of him, because we weren't competing. He was winning in the game of life. I was not. We would never meet on a competitive stage. He was simply being a good friend.

"Ok, I'm going to go confirm everything with Susan," he continued. He turned and left, and the door closed behind him.

My final two weeks amounted to little more than a farewell tour. Sean, one of the more senior associates, came by my office one day and asked if I had lunch plans. I did not, so we headed across the street to a converted firehouse called the Spotted Dog.

I rarely worked directly with Sean, likely because he did not enjoy my earlier propensity for turning in mangled assignments. But I rode with him once to a document storage center in Alabama for an on-site review, and during that trip, we had talked to pass the time. Thus, despite my limited contact with him at work, we always greeted each other in a friendly manner when we passed in the office halls. I was not taken back when he asked me to lunch, but I was unsure what the conversation would entail.

Once we sat down and put in our order, I started to see one reason why. He was nice and felt bad for me. My work had been poor, and his reviews had been damning.

"Now, where are you headed?"

"Cole Hyde."

"That's right. They are a smaller firm, right?"

"Yes, I think about fifty people, including the staff." I hoped this would be sufficient, since I didn't understand much more than that.

"Look, life at a big firm is pretty miserable. No one wants to do this forever. I know I don't. I think being at a smaller firm with more reasonable hours and less stress may be the only way to survive in this profession."

I nodded. I didn't believe him, but it seemed the courteous thing to do. I still wanted the big firm life, and his words were simply the product of his misunderstanding. He didn't know that I was still healing, that someday soon I would be back at full strength and would return to this forum with the ability to do the work. This was temporary, much like a woman who left on maternity leave.

He had chosen the pep talk delivered to the defeated by a pitying onlooker, but I was not finished fighting. I knew I would regain what I momentarily had to give up. Regardless, I did appreciate his polite approach. When he picked up the lunch tab over my protestations and we headed back to the office, I added him to the list of people I would miss during my sabbatical.

I seldom stayed the entire day during my final two weeks, but when I was there, I cleaned my office, read and responded to emails about Kevin's upcoming wedding, and arranged my final lunches with Chad and Susan.

We scheduled our goodbye lunch for Wednesday, since I knew I would leave directly after my exit interview on Thursday. We had our final Son's lunch the previous week, and since they were pressed for time, we went across the street to the Spotted Dog.

"It's good you escaped this place, but we're going to miss having you around the office," Susan began. "After you get settled, we need to make sure we make time to get together for lunch. I want to hear all about your new job."

Stories about Peyton and Jake circulated, I discussed my pathetic social life and potential dating opportunities on the horizon, and we tried desperately to avoid all mention of work. It was comfortable, even as the finality of the event hid in plain sight. We continued to pick at the food until, after glancing at his watch, Chad admitted they needed to get back, because he had to send the borrower his revisions by three o'clock. As the elevator opened, we said our professional goodbyes. I knew then that I wouldn't see them at work in the foreseeable future, but would keep in touch with them outside the office. I returned to my office and puttered around for a few minutes before I headed back home.

I slept well that night, but when my eyes opened in the morning, I felt another wave of regret, knowing it was officially my last day. Two hours after I got in to work, I met with Gina. The interview was a series of questions designed to assist the firm in developing work protocols to better retain employees.

"Did you feel that the group was structured so that you had opportunities for client contact?" she asked. "If you had questions about an assignment, did you feel like you could ask other members of the group for assistance?"

I formulated the honest answer in my head first.

"I didn't have much client contact, outside of the assignment registering a developer with the Veteran's Administration, but that was probably good, since I spent most of my time here so scared that I was about to piss myself. I felt like Chad May shielded me for as long as he could from the consequences of my unfortunate incompetence while he tried to teach me what I was doing, but seeing as I showed no ability to learn the most basic tasks imaginable, his efforts could not have saved me. I mastered the concept of saving a document to our computer system in December. You really don't have to worry about whether the firm was the reason for my struggles and this exit. It wasn't. You don't want to keep people like me, anyway."

Even then, I knew that the honest answer running through my head was inappropriate. This was an exit interview. The self-pitying monologues, which usually featured a fully stocked bar, remained internal and were held in the evenings—the guest list did not include the firm HR director. Plus, I did not want to burn any bridges in case I decided to return to this particular firm when I finished healing. I chose, instead, to go with a more subdued response.

"I had sufficient client contact, and Chad May and Susan Oliver did an excellent job of explaining everything to me." I hoped my vanilla answer would ensure that Chad and Susan received credit for their efforts. Still, since I didn't want them blamed for my shortcomings, I made sure to provide the necessary addendum. "The failures were of my own accord, and, without their help, I would have struggled even more."

I passed her my building entry card as I rose to leave.

"Thank you for your time, Neil. Good luck with your new job."

Mercifully released, I took the back stairs down a flight to my office and made my final tour of the floor to say my official goodbyes. After I completed the loop, I returned to my office and, sitting in my chair, I turned to face my wall of windows twenty-three stories above the city one last time. I knew I would miss the view. I headed to the exit, and the ding of the elevator bell let me know it was time to enter the one to my left and begin my descent. I would never return to these heights.

{chapter 25}

I rode home in silence, thinking about what was to occur. I thought maybe tomorrow would be the day I finally emerged from my cocoon and dazzled everyone. But there were too many contingencies for me to feel confident that this would happen, though I hoped it finally would.

Back at the apartment, readying myself for the following day, I knew most of my concerns were the garden variety issues anyone would worry about before beginning a new job. Did I remember where it was? I double-checked my route to the office to make sure. I set my alarm clock next to my bed and the alarm on my phone to guarantee my prompt arrival. Since my business casual wardrobe would no longer suffice, I took great care in assembling what I was to wear, setting out my black suit and a carefully chosen tie, which I then practiced tying so the knot would not resemble a misshapen softball.

After I completed these tasks, I reheated some Chinese takeout I had ordered the day before and mindlessly devoured it while I sat in front of my TV watching the previous day's Tivo'd PTI. When I finished, I threw my plate into the dishwasher and aimlessly wandered through my apartment picking up. I was out of things to do. So I headed to bed, even though it was only nine.

I couldn't lie still in bed. My mind would not turn off. The night was just beginning, but I was already panicked. I wouldn't be going in to my office on high the next morning. As I was tired of my failures, I hoped the change of employer would provide a welcome respite from my unending fear of termination, and my new location would allow me to thrive. I needed my efforts to finally result in success. Once this happened, I would calm

down and enjoy everything. I could achieve this in my new job.
No one knew about my wreck, which meant people would no
longer interpret random mistakes as a sign of deeper struggles.

This time, though, I didn't have a security blanket, and I
knew it. My old accomplishments could no longer save me
from my present failures. The partners would have expectations,
and if they were not met, I would simply be fired. I had no idea
if I would be able to do the work. It was so different from what
I had done before that they certainly expected a learning curve.
But what would I do if my mind continued to flat-line? The back
and forth continued unrelentingly, depriving me of the peace of
mind necessary for sleep. I tossed and turned, never slipping
fully out of consciousness until, too tired to patiently wait any
longer, I moved to the kitchen, grabbed a beer, and headed for
the living room. I would consume two more while watching
some syndicated show reruns before, my mind pummeled into
submission, I returned to my room and finally got to sleep.

The next morning, my alarm woke me at seven o'clock. After
a shower, I put on my freshly laundered suit and, after three
attempts, managed to make my tie look respectable. On my
way out to the car, I rehearsed my interpersonal strategy.

Mom had once again reminded me when we talked a couple
of nights before that my wreck was not something I needed to
share with everyone at every possible opportunity. But my life
made no sense without adding it. Where was I from October
until January? Why had I left Irwin Myers? Why didn't I
understand much about practicing law after being a lawyer for
over a year?

"When do people ask you those questions?" she had finally
asked.

They didn't ever ask. But they could.

"Why not wait until they ask, and then share?"

I was anticipating lines of questioning that would only
rarely occur. I was the only one defining me by my wreck. With

my move to Cole Hyde, there was finally an incentive to stop talking about it. My co-workers weren't going to ask why I left my old job, or, if they did, a stock answer would suffice. No one cared where I was during those missing months. I had already survived the interviews, so they no longer cared about the past and instead wanted to know about the present.

I was already limiting the story-telling as best I could, no matter how much I wanted to impress people with my recovery or explain away my failures. At my new job, it was my secret. These people would never meet the ones who had listened to the earlier stories. This world didn't need to know about it. I would stop the research into my condition. It was time for a fresh start.

Upon my arrival at my new place of employment, I parked in the visitors' section. The guard buzzed me in, and I headed to the third floor to begin anew. First came the perfunctory introductions to my new colleagues and, as is customary on the first day, everyone was friendly. I shook hands with anyone who greeted me in the hall, deliberately making eye contact and trying to exude friendliness. After the introductions, I walked down to my new office.

Upon entering, the view was hardly spectacular, but it was familiar, since I knew the area from living nearby. After pausing at my desk to collect myself, the second order of business was to create a series of mnemonics to help me remember at least some of the names. A few minutes later, I met with the office manager, Joyce, to take care of the administrative forms and to receive my key card, which assured me access to the building. Since it was a Friday, the office was slow, and though Alan briefly discussed one deal on which he was working, the day was predominantly dedicated to administrative matters. The office was soon empty, and I headed down to the elevator and out to my car. This journey, with all of its uncertainty, had officially begun.

{the detours}

The weekend offered a reprieve from the new. I holed up, preparing for my trip to Mobile for Kevin's wedding. My first full workweek would only be a four-day week, so it would be survivable.

Monday arrived, and I soon confirmed what Alan had already told me: I would be doing transactional work, as opposed to strictly real estate. I told myself that the promised diversity of assignments would keep everything fresh. This was going to work out just fine.

Even with my internal pep talks, my stomach churned due to my frayed nerves. I kept reminding myself that I only had to survive until Thursday. If I could make it through Thursday, I would be back in my element on Friday, socializing and carousing with people I knew.

The week flew by, and though I worked tirelessly at getting up to speed and my workdays extended well into the evenings, I hardly even noticed. Once I left the office, I was home within a few minutes, where a dinner of spaghetti sated my hunger. Even by the end of my abbreviated first week, I had quieted my uncertainty about how my work was regarded, something I was unable to do during the entirety of my tenure at Irwin Myers. No one knew. By Thursday, I had my weekend itinerary fully planned, my bags were packed and loaded into my car. That night, I finally slept well.

{chapter 26}

My arrival in Mobile was not greeted with an actual parade, but the first familiar face I saw at the hotel was sufficient, even without confetti-covered onlookers lining the streets . I had been back to the city only once since my wreck, but this particular trip was intended to revisit my distant past, not my recent detour, and other than a tennis tournament long since relegated to the dusty shelves in the furthest recesses of my mind, I had no memories of this town. My law school friends—those with whom I had shared my golden days of existence—promised the familiarity I longed for.

Upon arriving, I dropped my bag in the hotel room I would share with Joel and Craig, my law school friend who had just returned from his honeymoon when my wreck took place. The room had a queen bed and a pullout couch; I opted for the couch and situated my stuff accordingly. I jumped in a willing driver's car as we headed for the tux rental place to confirm everything fit, which thankfully it did.

Then we headed to the beach. Armed with SPF 45, my genetic pastiness, so painstakingly re-affirmed under the fluorescence of my daily office life, would not be my undoing. A greater menace was the cooler of beer that soon joined us, thanks to one of the groomsman, but in spite of my less than illustrious history with this beverage, I didn't fear it as much as I did the sun's relentless rays.

I joined a friendly crowd on the beach, begging some of the guests for beer, but I didn't know anyone particularly well, since these were mostly Kevin's friends from UGA. I remembered many of them from their weekend stops in New Orleans while I lived with Kevin, but some of them may have preceded my mid-year tenure in our law school house. Still, with the large collection of people around me, it was easy to pretend I knew everyone, unless I was informed otherwise.

Beer quickly circulated through the crowd of men, all only recently emancipated from the chains of school dreams, and still relatively fresh from the four or six or seven years of relative relaxation that preceded reality. I lifted a beer to my mouth and let its cool refreshment soothe me.

Joel arrived at the hotel about the same time I did and was part of the first landing party on the beach. Craig had to finish a half day of work and would join up later. Joel and I greeted one another with a handshake and a half-hug, notifying onlookers of our status as good friends. I hadn't seen Joel since my accident, but I was relieved to find nothing about our dynamic had changed.

"How's D.C.?" I asked.

"It's good. I've been playing a ton of tennis at my club. I play singles when I can, but I play doubles in a league. Most of the guys at the club are older, but some of them are still strong players. How about you? You playing much tennis these days?"

There was no talk of work, no reminder about what I couldn't do. We were two guys talking tennis, like we had in law school. And I stood there, the question only briefly hovering in front of us. I was so close to slipping back into my old clothes, and I didn't care if they fit. I wanted it so badly. I had an answer ready and I delivered it quickly, hopeful he wouldn't notice what had changed. I was different. I didn't know where I was going or how I would get there. But he let me pretend.

"I haven't had many opportunities to hit since I got to Atlanta. I brought my racquets. Thanks for reminding me about that, or I would have forgotten them. Do you want to find somewhere to hit this afternoon?"

"There is a park right down the street from the hotel," he told me. "Once Craig gets into town, we can all head down there."

Joel knew the UGA crew better than I did, and I tagged along behind him and was soon in the middle of the throng. Kevin held court, greeting everyone by name as he circulated the group on the beach, meandering through the crowd, inquiring how everyone was doing. It was his parade, and it was fun to watch him enjoy the moment. He smiled his pageant smile and wove through the onlookers like a politician in front of his constituents. He stopped in front of me, and we greeted one another again, in the same manner Joel and I had a few minutes before. The familiarity was comforting.

"How's everything going? Are you boning some new skank in Atlanta?"

Kevin's crudeness, reflected in his law school house reputation as Mr. Disproportionate Response, was generally on display when surrounded by his guy friends. I felt accepted, as our group's daily interaction around our law school friend group flooded back.

"Kevin, why did you leave your dish in the sink?"

"I was too busy boning your sister to worry about it."

I knew my role here was to play the straight man now. I could resume my role as No Filter Neil in a different setting.

"Things are going well. No new skank, but I'm always on the lookout. I started my new job last Friday."

"How's the job going?" he asked.

His follow-up question reminded me that we weren't in law school anymore. We lived in a world with jobs, where girlfriends became wives, where people traded in the dingy house rented with three friends that had a wall of televisions in the living room for a home in a respectable area of town and the corresponding mortgage. He didn't have all of this quite yet, but we were celebrating his first step this weekend.

Yesterday's comfort no longer existed today. I knew it was a good thing, and regardless of my reluctance or inability to move on beyond what used to be, I was happy to find him doing well. I pretended to dwell in the present, but my present wouldn't let go of my past.

"They don't have any idea who they have. The partner I work for thinks he stole one of the bright legal minds away from a big firm with promises of a shortened work week. My job is to become that guy before he figures out otherwise."

"Good luck with that. Don't forget, the rehearsal is at five. The directions to the church are in the packet in your room. After that, we are doing a crawfish broil at a place just down from the hotel."

The bridal party joined the groomsmen as well, but I knew none of them, so I sought out Rachel immediately, hoping to avoid any potentially awkward social interactions with her friends.

Her eyes lit up as we hugged hello. Rachel had seen me lying in a hospital bed at the trauma hospital, where she sat with Amy and everyone else when there was little remaining hope. She stopped in at my rehab facility on a trip to Augusta; when I was surrounded by unbelievably injured minds, she affirmed for me that people remembered me, not as a source of email text, not as a regrettably damaged person worthy of pity, but as a friend—a concept so foreign to my fellow inhabitants that she was the talk of the place for the remainder of that week. She had seen me and Amy at the beach the previous July 4th, Amy already fatigued after a month and a half of dealing with me and my realities. She and Kevin had invited me to witness the good in their lives when all I'd shared with her were my lows.

That flash in her eye, the look on her face as we briefly embraced, was not a product of anything I had done for her. She was happy that I could be a part of this event marking the official beginning of their lives together. I appreciated that they had included me, but after stumbling through an inadequate attempt to convey this, I realized I was without the ability to accurately express my feelings on the subject. I wished her well, and I retreated to the safety of the known.

Craig arrived at the beach and, after a little while, we headed back to the hotel to change into our tennis gear and find the courts. The woman at the hotel's front desk gave us directions to the courts, located in a nearby park.

While Craig was still the most athletic among us, he was the least experienced tennis player, and he was supposed to be the weakest player. Joel stood at the far end, while Craig and I shared the other side of the court. The ball in play, I channeled my successful tennis persona and crushed a forehand. It landed two feet out. My next shot, a slice backhand, ended up in the middle of the net.

I grew dizzier with each attempted shot. My beach consumption was not to blame, since I only had two beers, but my balance began to betray me anyway, and my tentative movements were insufficient to cover even my half of the court. We took serves. My first one was long, my second one in the net. The third one I failed to even make contact, as my racquet sliced through the empty air under the toss that remained too high for me to reach.

It was humiliating. My failures in front of the wheelchair-bound men during rehab were frustrating, but they had no point of reference, no idea from where I had fallen. I conveniently forgot that Joel only knew my tennis game from law school, when I hadn't played with any frequency for four years. The cursing became more necessary than breathing. I had to show everyone I knew how pathetic my display was.

"What the fuck!" I screamed.

"Another fucking shank?"

"Hit the ball on the fucking strings! Ninety-five fucking square inches and you keep hitting the fucking frame? What the fuck is this?"

"I wish you had fucking died, so I wouldn't have to see this, you worthless piece of shit."

The fun had died for me, so I mercilessly killed it for everyone else. This weekend was supposed to announce my return and the resumption of an unfinished trip. I knew it wasn't the main reason we were gathered there, but I felt as if it was an interesting subplot. Two people began their lives together while I resumed my old one. But this wasn't happening the way I had planned.

Craig and Joel finished their tie-breaker while I watched and, tired of tennis and my hissy-fits, we headed back to the hotel to get ready for the rehearsal. Craig was a groomsman, which entailed more work than Joel's and my roles as ushers.

Bride or groom? I could handle my job. Simply seat the guests appropriately, proceed in, and sit in my designated seat. No one would notice me for more than three minutes. For once, I found a task so basic I didn't think I could mess it up. But I was a little concerned about which arm I should offer the woman I was escorting. A frantic questioning of Joel provided an answer. He told me to offer my right. He thought this was the answer, and that worked for me.

The rehearsal commenced. After we finished the walk through, the minister said a few words about marriage, deemed the rehearsal a success, and the wedding planner delivered her demands regarding timeliness and confirmed we had all picked up our tuxes. We were then released to begin the evening. The restaurant was close to the hotel, and after a quick stop at the room, we headed back out to the dinner to commence the drinking.

I knew Kevin's UGA friends could drink, and I vowed to keep up, despite my well-earned reputation as a lightweight.

Each beer I downed brought me inches closer to that magical time in law school where I had lived just inside the periphery of fun due to my associates, many of whom were now in my presence and, skunk drunk, everything had worked out fine. I was the lazy, drunk, smart kid. I was well on my way to embracing the second adjective so frequently attributed to me. Perhaps this would remind everyone of the third.

The party continued after the rehearsal dinner, as the wedding party headed out to join the other people in town for the weekend. I made it to the next stops in body only, and though I undoubtedly said my hellos to Amy, and my other friends from law school who had made the trip to Mobile, my mind had stopped recording the evening's events and was no longer making significant contributions to my decision-making.

The next morning, I woke to the sound of my heartbeat in my head, confirming I was still alive and causing me to question whether I wanted to be. Something didn't feel right, even before my eyes fully opened. The first thing I noticed was that I was in the bed. This wouldn't have troubled me much, had I not somehow remembered the very end of the evening, which came to a close with me on the pullout and Joel and Craig in the bed. Something else didn't feel right. Before I could determine what it was, someone began pounding on the door. Craig grudgingly left the sofa and opened the door, to find Kevin there, grinning and barely able to contain his spastic energy.

I raised my head from the pillow to see who it was, squinting as I felt for my glasses on the table next to the bed.

"Are you still fucking naked?" Kevin yelled as he bounded into the room.

I gingerly lifted the sheet and peered below. That was the problem. I was buck naked. This was a startling revelation to wake up to, especially when paired with my horrendous headache. I quickly grabbed a pair of shorts out of my bag next to the bed and remedied the situation.

Kevin wouldn't shut up. His voice was already twice as loud as he usually made it, and his ordinary volume would have been too loud for my aching head. He kept gleefully repeating what he had announced upon his entrance. I knew that I would not be living this down anytime soon, if ever.

Though I understood why he was losing his mind, I was still confused about precisely what had occurred. The situation was clarified for all of us when Craig began to narrate the story of the previous night while Kevin giddily looked on. Apparently, I had gone to the bathroom in the middle of the night, and, after completing this rudimentary task, I shed my clothing and headed for the bed, where I went to sleep on top of the covers in between Joel and Craig. Craig discovered this almost immediately and scurried to the couch in horror. Joel remained on his half of the bed, and I moved to Craig's newly vacated side, where I managed to finally get under the covers.

Kevin couldn't contain himself. He suddenly was in possession of more material to make fun of me than he could ever fully use, though I knew he would try his damndest to do so. In many ways, I had given him the perfect wedding present. After the thank you notes were written, he wouldn't have any idea what I bought him, since I certainly wouldn't. This, he would remember forever.

He ran out of the room and down the hall to share with his other friends what he had learned. At that moment, absolutely mortified about what was circulating among the wedding party—just briefly—everything felt right. He wasn't worried about whether I could handle the mocking I would deservedly receive. He didn't care why I had gotten so drunk, since I used to get ridiculously drunk all the time in law school. He didn't want to further analyze the situation to uncover the source of my pain. He wanted to laugh uncontrollably at his friend who did something so stupid that failing to ridicule him would be unfathomable. He had no intention of kid-gloving me. We were friends, like we had been before, the kind who gave each other shit when the situation called for it.

We all ended up in Kevin's room, killing time before getting ready for the ceremony. I was the punch line of every joke at first, but the pace gradually slowed to one in three, then one in four.

"Watch the cornhole, guys," Kevin advised my roommates in between chuckles.

My initial discomfort was replaced with an appreciation for being included in the joke. Most of the onlookers probably saw me as the object of ridicule, but I viewed it as being an indispensable element of a shared experience. Craig, Joel and I did not appreciate the event's occurrence, but as a story, it was a source of mild embarrassment for me and great amusement to those not involved.

After the laugh-in in Kevin's room, I went back to my room, where I showered, shaved and assembled my tux. Miraculously, I once again found all of the necessary accessories and, as I boarded the bus for the church, I looked respectable. The photographer began taking the wedding pictures after our arrival, and while he assembled subgroups, I listened for him to tell me what group I belonged to. At Kevin's direction, I joined his picture with his ushers as well as a picture with the Tulane group.

After we finished the group photos, we took our positions in the church, and the first people began to arrive, and so our duties as ushers began. Upon my return from seating a nice couple that knew Kevin from his younger years, I saw Amy, who was talking with Joel.

"I heard you had a rough night last night," she said as I approached.

I tensed, but kept my sense of humor as best I could. "What straight guy hasn't always wanted to wake up and find himself naked in bed with a roomful of guys and know that he was sandwiched between two dudes earlier in the evening, then have an entire wedding full of people hear about it? I can now check that off my list."

It got a laugh, which was good enough for me, and Joel escorted her to her seat while I awaited the next contestant.

Finally, they lined us all up, and we proceeded into the church. The wedding went smoothly, and I watched the two of them begin the next phase of adulthood. They were happy. I was happy for them, and at the reception, with the aid of another full keg, I had plenty of help faking my own happiness in front of my ex-girlfriend and my other friends.

Midway through the reception, sitting at my table with my half-empty beer in front of me, I looked up at the room. The mood was appropriately festive, and everyone else had a beer in front of them, too. But tomorrow, after brunch, they would all return to their lives, whatever that specifically entailed, and would recount to coworkers and friends stories of their fun weekend in Mobile. And then they would go about their daily routine. None of my law school classmates wanted to return to their Tulane days except for occasional visits. They had moved on.

I was trying to cling to a past that no longer corresponded to the present. It wasn't just because I was no longer the same guy who left New Orleans for Aiken that August day. They weren't the same people who walked across the stage to accept their diplomas, either. I took another swig from my increasingly empty cup. I vowed to consider what this meant after I grabbed my next beer.

{chapter 27}

I returned to Atlanta, and the monotonous drone of my life resumed. After only a few months, I already knew my new job was not going well. I spent almost all of my waking hours at the office, trying desperately to gain the expertise that everyone expected me to have. Alan took me under his wing and tried to walk me through my assignments. The concepts made perfect sense as we talked about them, but by the time I exited his office, I remembered virtually none of the lesson he had shared with me a few minutes before. I had hoped to leave my baggage at Irwin Myers and start fresh. It was becoming clear to me that a fresh start was not going to fix what was wrong with me.

In a universe where I lacked solutions for my macro problems, my only hope was to tackle every small problem individually and in that way create a piecemeal path away from my predicaments. Unfortunately, though my issues had joined me at my new office, some of the tools I once used to cope with them were no longer available. The fountains of energy found on the twenty-third floor of my previous employer were nowhere to be found in this new office, and I started bringing in my own supplies. Soon I found myself in the checkout line of the Publix with a cart full of two-liter Diet Cokes. By three o'clock in the afternoon, a large empty bottle adorned my desk, and the naked ice cubes in the cup next to it promised no further help. My eyelids began to sag and my thoughts moved as if wading through knee-deep syrup. I still wasn't sleeping well, but I was in bed for over nine hours a night, and I didn't see any way I could remedy my fatigue on that end. Instead, I switched substances, moving on to Diet Mountain Dew; every sip of the glowing green substance reminded me of how unnatural this was, so I supplemented with Diet Red Bulls.

One day, in my attempt to meet a deadline, I worked through the night at the office, and as the sun began to rise around six-fifteen, I felt a paralyzing wave hit. I knew I only had a few more hours and then this project would be done. Like a distance runner with the finish line in sight, I felt a final burst of energy as I remembered how little there was left to complete. The jolt wore off two minutes later, and my eyes tried to give up. But I knew this was not an option, and despite feeling drained of energy, I forced my eyes open and headed across the road to Starbucks to pick up my first cup of coffee as a professional.

I entered the store, bleary-eyed and nauseous from lack of sleep, and cognizant that the prior evening's efforts would all be for naught should I prove unable to pull everything together in the final few hours. The fresh smell of coffee beans woke me enough for my fears to surface, even while all other activity remained dormant. I had always seen coffee as the nuclear option. If coffee would not remedy the fatigue problem, there did not seem to be a legal alternative. My career path necessitated all-nighters on occasion, and if I couldn't handle the hours with the use of legal stimulants like coffee, I couldn't work as an attorney. The cup of coffee I hoped to purchase was no longer just a cup of coffee.

The store was already humming with people when I entered, and I stood back and scanned their menu. When I finally moved into line, accompanied by the feeling of inevitable doom, I realized I was the only twenty-six-year-old in the United States who couldn't handle a Starbucks. All I wanted was caffeine, but I did not speak this language. What remained of my career seemed to hinge on whether or not I could figure out how to do something a twenty-year-old kid instinctively knew how to do and, should I complete this basic endeavor, whether this standard formula for surviving sleep deprivation would have the same effect on someone like me, who could barely survive an ordinary work day.

When my turn came, I stepped to the cashier and, reading the menu on the wall on the other side of the counter in the same stilted manner a touring American exchange student read his French from a pocket dictionary, I placed my order for a grande Café Americano. Shuffling through the crowd of determined people fighting off the fatigue from little Suzie's midnight sniffles, or a late night of chasing a special someone whose skirt had promisingly revealed flesh at the margins of lewdness, I made it to the counter, where a disinterested worker presented me with what I hoped would be salvation.

I trudged back across the street to my office with surprisingly less money but with a steaming cup of coffee contained in a cardboard-banded cup with the accompanying graphic depiction that informed everyone I had finally come to realize the importance of adulthood. After all of those experiments seeking the right aid to overcome my perpetually drained existence, I was betting not only the evening's efforts, but also my future, on the tried and true method of coffee. What had happened to me that I felt as if my entire life was to be decided by something as trivial as a cup of coffee?

I waited until I exited the elevator on the third floor and made it down to my office before I finally nervously lifted the cup to my lips. The effect was not immediate, but within the hour, my choice proved to be more effective than I had imagined possible. My mind still ran more slowly than I would have liked, but I finally felt awake. When I left the office at three that afternoon, after a surprisingly productive morning, I knew I had found my answer to the problem of fatigue. I bought a coffee machine that weekend, and every day thereafter, I was wide awake for my daily frustration.

Another solution in hand, I now prepped for my day with two cups of coffee and headed into the office with my well-insulated coffee pot in hand, providing an additional three cups over the course of the day. Although I had arrived at a solution for one of my issues, this remedy did not solve the litany of other problems I was experiencing, and my professional life remained troubling.

My naïve dream of using this position as a jump-off point to resume my big firm career was proving absurd, since I had struggled from the outset in my new position. My continued presence there was beginning to feel as unlikely as it had during my last tenure. Still, I lived at the office, straining with everything I had to not fail here as well, but my nerves were beginning to fray.

I tried to do what I could to calm myself down, returning to the one-time salvation of intramural sports. Once a week, I played softball with the UVA intramural softball team after work. On the scheduled day, I drove to the field. When I left my car, I felt certain this was the day I was destined to die, by way of an errant throw or a bad ball skipping off a rock in the infield and into my still-fragile face. Doom mercilessly tracked me everywhere, and there I was defenseless. Many of my previous physical issues persisted, and I could not track the ball in the air without becoming dizzy. Luckily for me, I also could not accurately throw, and Jamie played me at catcher, a position usually reserved for your worst girl in co-ed leagues, since it did not require mastering fundamentals like catching or throwing under pressure. I was one of the league's worst catchers.

Saturdays, I played kickball with the same group. It was an excuse to stand in a field and drink beer. I didn't think it was possible to be bad at this. But when I stepped in to kick, poised mid-stride on one leg just before I made contact with the ball, my balance abandoned me and I left a ball dribbling down the third base line, guaranteeing me a hit and unrelenting taunting from the other team, who were convinced I had intentionally "munted," the term used for male bunting, which was the social equivalent of wetting oneself in high school.

Once safe from shame and well-hidden in the field, every time the batter began his or her stride toward the bouncing rubber ball, I fervently prayed the resulting kick would not send the ball in my direction. No matter where I played, at least once a game, it inevitably drifted toward the space I occupied. While my teammates raced toward me, trying to make the play before I muffed it, the ground shifted below my feet and my head began to swim as the unsteady cameraman showed me the arching red ball destined for my arms. Just as it arrived and my teammate pulled up short, I grew nauseous, and the ball bounced off my chest or landed a few feet behind me. They moved me to catcher.

I had played along in life initially, beating everyone to deliver the punch line about my pathetic efforts, and I had laughed loudest to show I was in on the joke, too. I could remind myself that the situations were funny to an outside observer, whether I was looking into the face of a disgusted date or being reassured by an annoyed teammate after that red rubber ball careened into the outfield. I tried so hard to outwardly maintain a sense of humor that I didn't actually possess. All while I seethed inside.

Then the day arrived that I could no longer even fake my laughter. My hobbies had become little more than reminders that I was terrible at everything. People had once wanted me on their team; now I could see the groan of my teammates as I arrived. My continued presence was tolerated by most but enjoyed by no one.

When I left the office in the evening, except on softball nights or occasional nights when Jill invited me out with her friends, I headed back to the apartment and moped about everything. It wasn't fair. It just wasn't fair. My promising career was over. I wasn't athletic. I had a dating life that vacillated between non-existent and unsuccessful. I was worse off in every way than I had been twelve months before. Why wasn't I healing? While I was still in the hospital, I at least had potential. Since then, I had become the personification of failure. My phone conversations continued the pattern of the dark days.

"Please stay positive. It is going to get better."

"No, it's not, Mom. I've been working my ass off for over two years, and my life is terrible. I can't live like this. My memory still doesn't work right. I think I'm going to be fired at work. I can't remember a day of work during my entire time in Atlanta when I didn't think I was about to be fired. I still have next to no friends. I'm bad at everything I try to do. I cannot fucking handle this."

"Calm down," she told me. "There is no reason to get yourself all worked up. Just relax, get a good night's sleep, and tomorrow will be better."

"No, it won't," I responded, my voice rising with frustration. "Every day is worse than the day before. Every day, I've woken up and pretended that everything is going to be fine. And every single fucking day, by the time I get home, I know nothing is okay."

"Neil, watch your language! I'm not going to listen to you while you sit around feeling sorry for yourself. Go to sleep, and I will talk with you tomorrow."

I defiantly laid down in my bed. I deserved to feel sorry for myself. I was a dead man walking. My defiance collapsed with the rest of me as the caffeine wore off, and I drifted off to sleep.

The next morning, my jaw ached, but it was different from the pain I had experienced earlier during my time in Atlanta. I washed down two ibuprofen with my second cup of coffee and headed in to work. The following morning, my jaw still hurt. I examined my mouth in the mirror, trying to figure out if there was a protruding wire or something visible that could explain this, even though the pain was nowhere near sharp enough to signify a puncture wound. Again, the pills went down and I headed for the door.

After waking up the third morning with my jaw again throbbing, I knew that the painkillers were only an exercise in denial, and I needed to take further steps to remedy the problem. When I arrived at my office the next morning, I called an in-plan dentist two blocks away and scheduled an appointment for the following day.

I arrived at the dentist's office at nine the next morning, once again experiencing the familiar facial discomfort. I had used this same dentist a few weeks earlier to have my teeth cleaned, so I was familiar with him. He entered the room in the manner of a dentist trying not to spook his terrified patient and greeted me with a friendly hello.

"Hi, Neil. Sorry to see you back so soon. What seems to be the problem today?"

He was familiar with my plate issues from our first visit, but I wanted to make sure he remembered my facial issues before presenting him with the problem.

"Well, I don't know if you remember, but I am the guy who had that car wreck where they had to put all of those plates in my face."

"I remember you telling me about it. Are you having some sort of issue with one of the plates now?"

"I honestly don't know. My jaw throbs every morning after I wake up. Some of the pain seems localized in the jaw orbital where they screwed it together. Maybe the screw is poking through into something else? I don't know."

He inspected my mouth, and once he left the room, one of his dental hygienists stayed behind and led me to another room to take some x-rays of my mouth. Afterwards, I returned to the first room, and when he came back into the room, he was holding up the x-ray pictures.

"I'm not seeing anything here. When I was looking at your teeth, I noticed some wear on your back molars, which seems to indicate that you are grinding your teeth at night. This is a common problem that I see, especially among people with stressful jobs, and being an attorney certainly qualifies as stressful, as I'm sure you can attest to. People who are under a lot of stress will unconsciously grind their teeth while they sleep. It explains the jaw pain. I am going to fit you with a mouth guard that I want you to wear at night. I'll give you a temporary one until the permanent one comes in. Wear it, and see if it helps. If it doesn't, we'll re-evaluate the situation."

I left his office, bewildered, and headed back to work. I already had enough problems, and now I was creating psychosomatic ones. It wasn't reassuring to me that this was a common problem among professionals in high stress jobs. Although convenient to blame, my job was only one factor contributing to my anxiety.

My inability to successfully cope with most of my problems had officially become a problem unto itself. My workday began, and I promised myself today would be different. I climbed out of my car and headed into the building.

Just relax, I thought.

{chapter 28}

The mouth guard served its purpose, and by the next week, I was pain-free. Unfortunately, this simply treated the symptom, not the core reasons behind my discomfort. It was becoming more and more clear to me, and in all likelihood, to my employers as well, that I wasn't working out at my job, despite my best efforts.

I trudged through my day, searching for chances to connect with people, resorting to the same failed strategies as before. I ate lunch with Chad and Susan as often as I could, though our lack of geographic proximity and our busy schedules limited these opportunities to once every two weeks or so. I dropped in to talk with my next-door neighbor at work, but she was busy and had a life outside the office that she was eager to return to at the end of the day, so she had no interest in lengthening her time at work by chatting with a coworker about his kickball travails. I grabbed occasional lunches with another coworker, but otherwise, my day was comprised of me working on an assignment, turning it in, and then sitting in my office, terrified that I had once again bungled it.

Mid-summer, Alan announced that an attorney, George Cooke, would be joining our team from South Carolina. I had done my best to forget that I was obligated to take the three-day South Carolina bar in February, but unlike the information I tried to remember but didn't retain, this nugget seemed to stick, and it had continued to worry me. Alan's announcement felt like an ominous sign. He was bringing in someone to take care of work he had once intended for me once I passed the South Carolina bar. But since I was aware of how unlikely my passage was, I was more relieved than threatened, and the first day George was in the office, I went down the hall to introduce myself, hoping to begin a camaraderie with someone else in the office. I needed the safe zone I had left behind with Chad and Susan.

Our first meeting was somewhat brief. We exchanged pleasantries. His mother still lived in Beaufort, and I talked about my family's frequent trips to Charleston. We had initiated a conversation about how great Charleston was when Alan's booming voice called for George to come to his office, so I headed back to mine to work through my latest assignment. The next day, George stopped by my office.

"You up for grabbing a beer tomorrow after work? Renee and I need to finish some unpacking tonight, but then I need a beer. Do you know a good place around here? I'm thinking there has to be a pub nearby."

"There is a place called Fados on Peachtree across from the ESPN Zone," I told him. "We can check it out, if you're up for it. It's part of a chain but is designed to feel like an Irish pub. It's dark as hell and there is usually a Premier League soccer game or a rugby match on, so it's a good change of pace from the other bars around here."

The next evening, with a Bass in my hand and a Guinness in his, we both began to unwind from our days. At first we talked about the office, but by the second beer, we had moved on and were discussing the perks of living in a big city like Atlanta. He was also a huge sports fan, and by the end of the evening, we concluded that we would find a time to check out the Braves before the end of the summer.

"I need to get back home to Renee, who is probably wondering where I am," he explained as he rose to his feet. "She wanted me to see if you would be interested in coming over for dinner sometime soon."

"That sounds good to me," I answered. "I'd love to meet her. I'll take a look at my calendar tonight and see what works for me. See you tomorrow."

I left the bar and headed for home. As I finished the short walk, I realized I had, quite possibly, befriended my replacement, though I knew it might once again be my paranoia. Regardless, from my perspective, the firm had conveniently brought in a guy who seemed like he was usually up for a beer, was into baseball, and who took the pressure off me to pass the South Carolina Bar.

In an act of self-preservation, I had instinctively averted my eyes from the unattainable career goals I previously created, and the foundation for something larger than my job was slowly being established. I made it to dinner at George and Renee's the next week, and she was both incredibly sweet and a terrific cook. In the years to come, my friendship with George would continue to grow. We would go to Braves games, I would be in their wedding and we would go in together on Hawks partial season tickets. They would become some of my good friends in Atlanta. My job, always so central to my existence, was still informing much of my life, but its once dominant legacy was transitioning from a realm that defined me in totality to one that provided chance introductions while it attempted to shun me.

Another woman, Taylor, who was friends with Jill from law school, lateralled in to a position in Atlanta from her former job in New York. New to town and without a built-in social network at her disposal, she warmed to my offer of friendship, and we began grabbing dinner or drinks with some degree of frequency as well.

With these newest friends, I was adding even more people to my life who remained on track professionally, and I had the opportunity to see what success looked like, often in the same arenas where I had tried and failed. I would not initially understand their insecurities with their own work performance or know of their frequent weekends in the office until our friendships developed more fully over the years that followed. But even with different career trajectories, I could now count these people as friends. Between my new friends and my continuously failing pursuit of UVA intramural greatness, some days I was so busy that I forgot to be miserable about work.

Even with my improved life outlook, by the middle of October, work was going poorly enough that I began to accept that this job too, would end badly. Mom was tired of listening to the same complaints, and I was tired of being scared. I was not going to be able to right this ship, and though I promised myself I would not stop trying on the off chance I could salvage something, I began to prepare for the inevitable crash. My weaknesses would define me, whether I accepted it or not. I started hoarding paychecks. I could cook and subsist on spaghetti and salad, so I stopped eating out and ate cheap pasta, which I knew how to make. And I contacted Wendy and scheduled a time to resume my quest for the perfect, attainable job.

As I resumed my work with Wendy, her focus remained on what I wanted, and she encouraged me to explore what made me happy. She still hoped to pair me with the career best suited for me, and she seemed hopeful that this latest discontent with my current career destination would convince me to alter my approach.

Unfortunately, I still stubbornly refused to consider new criteria in my search.. I was still focused on finding a job from which I could not be fired, and as I was learning just how unqualified I was for most jobs, job security was the only factor that I could look for.

Struggling to come up with an answer to her straightforward inquiries about what I wished to do, I mentioned that the non-profit sector, with its potentially more relaxed schedule and grateful clients, could be something of interest. I doubted they would fire people with any degree of frequency in this profession. And with that, I stumbled back into who I now was.

Wendy pondered her connections within the non-profit world and remembered that one of her other clients was a member of a group that did volunteer work with the Shepherd Center, and she put me in touch with the woman, Alyssa, via email. During our first email exchange, Alyssa informed me that there was an upcoming meeting with the group, called the Shepherd Center Junior Committee. The Junior Committee was a group of young professionals that raised money to fund therapeutic recreation projects and programs for residents of the Shepherd Center. This was done through a large fund raising effort called Derby Day—a huge Saturday party organized by the committee that revolved around the Kentucky Derby. She forwarded a link and promised that I would learn more about the group and its mission at the next meeting later in the week.

Alyssa's subsequent email provided the exact time and location of the meeting, and I made sure to attend. What began simply as an initial job search began transforming into something more significant almost immediately. Work was again rejecting me, and I would quickly come to see volunteer opportunities like this as a potential solution to my feeling utterly useless, a way to explore this world prior to applying for positions with a non-profit.

But in this instance, what was most appealing was the chance to use whatever aptitudes I still had to help the residents of a facility for which I was once eligible. I hadn't wanted to return to the subject that taunted me daily, I wanted it to disappear; but since this was not an option, I could help everyone else until it went away.

I arrived at the first meeting as early as possible and found the parking lot, which was situated among a cluster of buildings a few blocks up the road from my office. I had twenty minutes to spare when I emerged from the parking deck. But as I surfaced from the garage, looking at the numbers on all the buildings, I didn't see the building in which the meeting was being held. I wandered aimlessly among the multistory structures, but never found a building bearing the number I was searching for. I felt panic begin to rise, and with it, shame. This wasn't daunting. I just had to find the building and go in for a volunteer meeting, that was all. I was already struggling, even with this basic task.

I felt stupid and useless after a long day of feeling stupid and useless. Maybe I would drive home and go to the bar up the street and get a beer. I didn't need this frustration. I was completely worked up by the time I spotted a group of younger people dressed in professional-looking garb and asked a trailing member if this was the site for the meeting. It was. So I joined the herd.

It was an auditorium full of people who knew each other. We all wore nametags, in case anyone wanted to converse with someone outside the group of people they knew from college or last year's committee. I met up with Alyssa and her boyfriend before the meeting, and as we took our seats, the meeting began and everyone announced their name and undergraduate institution.

I began to understand what I was witnessing almost immediately. This was a group of young people who liked to have fun, and they were channeling that energy to benefit a cause. I certainly respected their desire to create such an organization, and I wanted to be a part of it, but I knew right away there were core problems with my participation. I hadn't been able to have fun since my wreck, and it was one of the group's underlying purposes. Also, my sudden bout of silence had not facilitated conversation with the strangers around me as effectively as I had hoped it would. I needed self-confidence that I did not possess before I could approach them and begin the basic task of meeting these new people. Greeting others with a friendly "hello" never occurred to me as an option. I considered only possibilities in which my accident played a role.

As the meeting wore on, I silently explored alternatives to my meek approach. Instead of sitting quietly, should I attend the happy hour that night? Maybe sit at the bar and explain over a beer to a group of people I had met shortly beforehand that I joined up because I was trying to justify my existence—my relative good fortune—by helping others who had suffered the same sorts of calamities but lost use of their legs or were severely handicapped as a result? How quickly would that kill everyone's buzz? How many seconds into my story would I be before I looked like the prick who was begging for attention when nothing was wrong with me, especially when compared to those for whom we were raising money—people who were facing far more daunting challenges and still had the optimism necessary to embrace life and the dedication to will themselves onto the national wheelchair fencing team? How would I explain that I needed to receive additional credit for being there, how my presence was more noteworthy than the other volunteers, without coming off as a terribly flawed person? The meeting came to a close, and people began to file out.

"Are you going to the happy hour?" Alyssa asked.

"No, I need to get back and take care of some things," I lied. "It was nice to meet you both. I am definitely interested in joining up with this, though, so keep me posted about the meetings."

I returned to my apartment, having spent my evening listening to people talk about others who suffered from brain and spinal cord injuries while sitting hidden in front of them; I knew I had connected more completely with the victims, the people who appeared on the slides without nametags, than I had with the well-meaning, well-labeled individuals who viewed them. I felt as if an important genealogy involved those with whom I shared no blood ties.

{the detours}

That night, sitting in my living room, I resumed my investigations into traumatic brain injury before bed. I was no longer a patient with untrained eyes trying to read medical texts in a rehab facility. I was a lawyer trying to understand his condition. The difference was more than semantics. Almost two years had passed. I could figure it out now.

The Internet was a predictably pathetic neurologist, but I could afford its rates, and though I returned little of interest my first night, persistent searching over the next couple of days disclosed some useful information. The articles Google provided generally focused on whether a brain injury had occurred and what the symptoms were.

I already knew I had a traumatic brain injury, so these were of little help to me, but the symptoms described me perfectly. I ticked them off as I went down the list: weakness in one or more limbs, sleep difficulties, sense of spinning, loss of memory, loss of balance, headache, and dizziness. I wasn't alone. These things described me, but they also described others. It wasn't my fault.

None of the articles could promise a timetable for recovery. In fact, further review of articles could not even confirm if a complete recovery was possible. Some articles indicated that it was, but most suggested that though the injured person could get close, he or she would never quite attain one hundred percent of who he or she had once been. I needed about ninety percent, so outside of the overarching worries of never being whole, I thought that the expected upper range was sufficient. Lack of a concrete timeline made me nervous, but this was the best I could find for free.

I revisited the articles again and again, and began focusing on the symptoms. Anxiety and nervousness? That explained the jaw pain I had just fixed with the help of a mouth guard, but I worried all through law school—I worried so much that I almost walked out of the bar exam. Depression? My morbid life outlook had lately been coming into focus, but despite living a charmed life before, I had always found a way to mope about things, from adolescence through college and even law school, sometimes to the point of becoming self-destructive. The clarity I believed my investigation would provide was not present. Maybe it was my fault. Or maybe self-doubt was a symptom not listed.

Furthermore, the articles were conjecture. I could spot it on the third or fourth reading. No one understood these problems, at least not fully. My ability to comprehend what they prescribed was not the issue. They didn't fully understand what they were talking about. They couldn't anticipate all of the symptoms. They could not accurately guess the victim's recovery. They spoke in vagaries, medical jargon disguising their ignorance. In the end, what they offered was no better than the insights provided by Miss Cleo.

Still, after retunring home from my daily disappointment, my nightly searching continued. A few evenings into my research, discouraged by what I was uncovering, I had decided to move on to a more suitable time investment, a complete escape, like my fantasy football roster. But just before I gave up for the night, I stumbled across a website dedicated to brain injury survivor support groups. There was one nearby at Emory, led by clinical psychiatrist Dr. Louise Cording. I hoped these people would understand what I was going through. I noted it on my calendar and planned on attending the next meeting.

I left directly from work the evening of that month's meeting to allow as much time as possible to reach the location where it was being held. After I parked my car in the gated lot, I entered the front of the building. The security guard who greeted me assured me that my car was fine where it was parked and directed me to the room on my left. I had no idea what to expect.

When I entered, Roger immediately walked up to me and introduced himself. He was friendly in an "aw-shucks" type of easygoing manner, and he mentioned he had been coming to the group for a while. I immediately noticed his earnestness, and as the evening progressed, I watched his ability to convey selfless empathy to those around him, not begging any of us to acknowledge, even when it was his turn to share his past, his own hurt that allowed him to understand. A couple, who also seemed to be one of the driving forces behind everything, also came up to me, introduced themselves, and welcomed me to the group. When Dr. Cording arrived, we all took our seats in a circle and began discussion.

I was terrible at remembering people's names, so the idea of meeting this many new people at once was daunting, but like the Shepherd Center meeting, everyone's shirt was adorned with a handwritten nametag we had filled out upon entering.

"No one here is very good at remembering names," Roger joked.

We all went around the circle and introduced ourselves, and everyone told why they were there. Some had had strokes of varying degrees of severity, and some had had head traumas that had disrupted their lives, impeding motor reflexes, making walking more difficult, and in some cases making continued permanent employment close to impossible. Dr. Cording was there to facilitate a discussion where they could all find strength and answers from their collective experiences—where we could find strength and answers from our collective experiences.

By the time the introductions had finished, I knew I belonged. These people understood. They knew what it was like to be an amnesia patient. They knew how frustrating everything became. They knew what it was to live with a condition that no one could quite explain to you, that no one could tell you would someday go away, or even that it was going to be like this forever. They knew the taste of uncertainty, how no meal, regardless of its grandeur, could mask its flavor, how it overpowered the sweetness of the birthday cake icing, how it always lurked in the back of your mind, never to be vanquished. They knew.

Yet I also knew that I had a horrible advantage over the other people in that circle. No one could see my injury unless I chose to show it. I suffered from its effects, but not with the same severity. I could see mine in my eyes in my bathroom mirror in the morning, in the fatally flawed document that I passed across my desk to the partner, and in my ever-burning self-loathing. But no one else could see the impetus for this. They knew I wasn't right, but I might even some day learn how to manipulate how I was perceived.

My fellow group members didn't hold it against me, not for even a moment, that I had won what should have been a reprieve to any of them at the end of their daily struggles, but that I still couldn't figure out how to enjoy my lucky break. I should have loved them for their selflessness, but I was too busy. I was already worried about the fact that I didn't fit perfectly here either, that I would forever be a man without a country.

"I hope that you will come back for our next one," Roger said to me as I walked out the door of the room.

I don't know if he could see my relief, already becoming secondary to the new anxiety, but I suspect he heard it in the softness of my decisive response.

"I'll see you next month," I told him.

{chapter 29}

The inevitable, even if ignored, remains on course. The dread built, and though I quieted it by keeping busy and subdued its effects with mouth guards and Unisom, it was never too far from my mind. One Friday morning in December, when my alarm went off, I awoke nauseous and had a pre-breakfast encounter with my toilet. Work had slowed, so I called in sick, hoping a day of rest followed by a weekend in would make me whole. Delaying my day of reckoning was not sufficient. By Monday afternoon, I was unemployed.

I was at Fados, my Fados. The Irish bar veneer greeted me when I entered. I was soon at the bar, and there was a beer I had not paid for in front of me. George joined me, and so did Travis, a work friend who had begun the same time as I had. The beer, my beer, would not suffer the ignominious fate of its former companion in the keg, now sitting down the bar from me in front of a demonstrative guy and his female companion, ignored and warming in its half-full glass.

Mine disappeared as rapidly as those Bud Lights at two in the morning had at F & M's bar in New Orleans. Those New Orleans nights may not have left memories even by that following day, but the morning conferences with my roommates were full of stories of yesterday's idiocy, and we had always started fresh a few hours later, no worse for wear, temporary headache aside. I thought that would work here as well. A wake for my career tonight was the first step. I would get up tomorrow morning and laugh about how stupid it had all been and start over.

"Dude, you kissed a girl's hand last night. She was skeeved out."

"You remember that assignment you couldn't figure out? Man, that partner was pissed."

Tonight was time to complete the cycle of stupid, so I could reminisce tomorrow and begin it all again.

"I haven't told anyone here, since I was trying to start over, but the reason I couldn't figure things out was that my memory doesn't work right. I had a really bad car wreck two and a half years ago. I was supposed to die, and I had to relearn how to walk and everything. My memory still isn't right."

I could tell this story in my sleep, and the beer in no way impeded my ability to emphasize the known details to show how dire it had been, and The Excuse was delivered perfectly, with all of its flourishes.

Die, mutha fuckas, die.

Relearn how to walk—TO WALK.

And I was expected to become an attorney after that? I had no short term memory and not much of a long term memory, either. It wasn't my fault.

The glass was empty again, but the bartender had not strayed far. He knew what kind of night this was for me, and he knew this was a Monday night for the bar. Everyone else had jobs to get back to. My party of three was the biggest thing going, and he didn't care what the theme of the evening was. He was simply the caterer.

"What they had you doing wasn't easy, either." Travis said. He had bought in.

"Wow, man, I wouldn't have guessed," George asserted reassuringly. "That is amazing. You're doing great."

He had hit his mark perfectly. The plate demonstration followed.

But they had work tomorrow, so the party began to disperse. About an hour after our arrival, Travis offered some words of encouragement and then departed to meet up with some other people with whom he had a prior engagement planned. George offered to take me home a couple of hours later, and knowing I had twelve of my friends in my refrigerator, I accepted.

He shuttled me down to my apartment at the bottom of the hill and let me out. I walked inside and set the alarm for noon. I needed to start packing for my Vegas trip. There was no reason to stick around here. There was nothing I wanted to see here, and Vegas held plenty of interest for me. I would have the chance to see Shawn again, since we were celebrating his return from his first tour in Iraq. And I hadn't seen Keith McCray, a friend I grew up with in Aiken, since his wedding. I killed two more while I sat in bed, before the curtain dropped with the lights still on.

The trip was only a week away, and since I already had my plane ticket, formalized plans to see friends and money budgeted for it, this seemed like an entirely justifiable expenditure. As for my tomorrows, my mind was as useless as that of a lobotomized frog prepared for dissection, which prevented things from hurting too badly. I wouldn't feel a thing. Everything would be fine. I needed to relax, and Las Vegas seemed to be the perfect venue to promote this strategy.

pulling off the road

{chapter 30}

A couple of days after I'd started preparing for Vegas, I was situated in my aisle seat, flying away from my problems. The plane ascended to its cruising altitude, and I rushed to open the book I had bought, Doyle Brunson's Super System: A Course in Power Poker. Not a moment could be lost. I needed to finish mastering poker during the three-hour flight. My eyes danced across the page. They didn't need to be confined by a ruler anymore and, alive with the excitement of an adventure in Vegas, they flirted with each word only briefly before flitting to the next phrase. There was knowledge to be captured, or at least be introduced to, and not a moment could be wasted. The thin pages taunted me, my left thumb's clumsiness slowing my proficient eyes, until I began depending solely on my right hand's dexterity. I had seen Rounders. I remembered some of my law school poker nights. I would dominate the tables. I was holding the book of knowledge, and with my earmarked funds, I would be untouchable. For one weekend, I had found my purpose.

The plane touched down after the long flight, and I was in Vegas, that beautiful land of today's temporary dreams and tomorrow's hangovers. I arrived in the day, and select veterans of last night's battles were tottering out of their temporary casino shelters or evening companion's abode and mixing with the innocence of the new arrivals. The neon's draw was somewhat repressed by the natural light that burdened those unfortunate souls who were suddenly awake to the consequences of last night's choices, but muted, artificial cheer still greeted the next group of eager tourists. The cold of the desert evening was trying to burn off, and I entered the casino to wait for Shawn's arrival from Hawaii.

The casino offered no respite from the overpowering sensory overload foreshadowed by the surrounding town. From the outside, my accommodations were a pyramid with a Sphinx guarding the entrance. The sun was not on the guest list and would not be admitted, but no one would miss it. The wall in front of me separated the check-in desk from the rest of the casino, and I perched at the back wall, bags in hand. A few minutes later, our choreographed plan was complete: Shawn stood in line with Chris, who was his fellow Navy officer from Hawaii. I already knew Chris from UVA. With that, the weekend began.

Shawn and Chris were dutifully admitted. I joined them, and we took the glass elevator up to our room to drop our bags. We paused for a few minutes to outline the weekend plan. Shawn was a planner. I was a follower. He talked, I nodded. Chris wanted desperately to gamble and didn't care about the plan.

"Brandon and Aaron will get in soon."

I knew Brandon from my days hiding in Pensacola at Shawn's place during the numerous hurricane warnings and optional evacuations that took place in my third year of law school in New Orleans. I knew Aaron from when he and Shawn lived together at Virginia.

"Keith and Natalie should be here by this evening. I'd like to go to the Cirque show tomorrow night. Other than that, there are a couple of other casinos I would be up for checking out. I'd like to go to the Hard Rock Casino, but you don't have to do that."

The expected personnel were a hodge-podge collection of my past friendships. Keith and I grew up in Aiken together. I had attended his and Natalie's wedding the December after my wreck, a wedding I was supposed to be in but ended up only observing, since they were nervous that I wouldn't learn to walk in time to participate.

Even though the timing of their appearances could not be pinpointed to an exact second, it was comfortable having the familiar around me. I knew Keith would be occupied with his wife, and the Navy guys, too desperate to celebrate their temporary emancipation from the order of their jobs to be stationary for long, were hard to pin down once they all got in, but that didn't matter to me. I could stop worrying. Nothing too terribly bad could happen here. I was surrounded by people I knew, who would be looking out for me, albeit in shifts, whether they consciously wanted to or not. I headed to the tables to make some money.

"I've been reading that Doyle Brunson book, and I think I've started to understand how to play Hold 'Em. He points out the game isn't about your cards, but how to read your opponents and how to bet against them. Since I think I understand that now, I'll be able to bluff more effectively and move people out, based on the flop. You have any interest in joining me at one of these tables?" I asked Shawn.

"I'll play a couple of hands, but I want to play Craps in a few minutes, then maybe some Blackjack."

We wandered to a nearby casino where we picked the cheapest table available and sat down. I bought in for $200 and put Doyle's plan into action—what I remembered of it, anyway. The most important feature of the table was the roving drink girl, and Shawn and I had cocktails in front of us by the second hand. The alcohol did not distract from my strategic play—it merely focused me further. The longer I stayed at the table, the more free drinks I would get. It was the short term incentive for my success that guaranteed I paid attention until the chips started piling up.

If my cards weren't suited or face cards, I tossed them. I observed how everyone played, watching to see how they bet.

I was focused. Shawn played a few hands, then cashed out and exited the table to find another game he could amuse himself with. I would catch up with him after I won a few hands and got bored here.

Very quickly, I discovered three main problems with my strategy. First, there was such turnover at the table that I couldn't keep track of who was who, and I never had the time to learn how anyone played. I couldn't remember if the guy across from me was the old guy I'd sat down with or someone new. The short guy who took the pot on the river on the last hand—was he the one who folded previously when someone raised the blind? I couldn't tell. The frat kids turned over every three minutes.

The second problem was that a week of reading Brunson's book and one airplane cram session had not imparted on me all of the wisdom of Texas Hold 'Em that his book had promised. My strategy was fragmented and faced with nearly identical situations, the courses of action I took varied wildly.

The third and, I told myself, the most important problem, was that I was playing low limit Hold 'Em, and the book was designed for no limit Hold 'Em. I struggled to move people out of the hand. Even with my judicious mucking of hands from the outset when I didn't like my cards, the stack of chips in front of me melted away quickly, as my high pair kept losing out to two lower pairs from the opposing players.

I was down to the last of my chips, but I was sitting to the left of the dealer, so I was the last one to play this hand. I would have the opportunity to see how everyone else was going to play before betting. I held a suited king and a jack, and when it checked around to me, I raised the blind. One guy dropped out, but everyone else came with me. The flop showed a king but nothing else of note. It checked around and I raised it, but again, everyone else called my bet. The turn eliminated the possibility of a straight or a flush. I raised the pot, and everyone called. The river was an inconsequential six. After it was checked around to me the final time, I threw all but one of my remaining chips.

I didn't feel very confident when two of the four remaining people came with me. One of them could have kings with a higher kicker. One of them could have pocket kings and be playing three of a kind. I felt like anyone with rockets would have bet them heavily, so I wasn't as scared of those, since I thought a low limit guy with pocket aces would become too excited and raise the hand at every opportunity.

We all turned over our cards, and at first glance, I knew I had won the large pot sitting in front of me. No one else was holding a face card. I smiled victoriously. Doyle Brunson had done me right. The pot had to be over $100, a killing for me at this table.

The guy two seats to my right let out a shrill cry.

"Yeah! Look at that! I won it on the last card! I love Vegas!"

I looked more closely at his cards. He had an unsuited three and six. He had beaten me on the river, playing a hand he had no business playing. I had played this particular hand like you were supposed to. With only a pair of threes, he had kept foolishly throwing money after my bets, which I made intending to run people with his low cards out of the hand. And he won it on the river for being dumb enough to hang around.

This was funny and educational, or it should have been. Sometimes the system just didn't matter, and pure chance dictated the results. What could have more clearly demonstrated this life lesson than what had just occurred? But even if this were the moral, I was also deliberately trying to apply a system I didn't fully understand to the wrong game, so my approach was flawed, regardless of what anyone else chose to do. Both of our approaches were "wrong," and the drunk guy who was living in the moment beat me. His strategy, as haphazard and ridiculous as I perceived it to be, was effective for him, even if he had lost. He was having fun. My focus on the end result robbed the entire game of all enjoyment.

Still, in my mind, he should not have won that hand. Since one of us had to win, I believed that I was somehow more deserving, and I sat stewing in my seat even as the dealer cleaned up the cards on the table. What had just occurred was not amusing to me, nor would it teach me anything. I focused instead on my victimization at his hands—I had been wronged yet again, and I deserved better. I tossed my last chip to the dealer as a tip, and stormed off to find my friends.

I first came upon Shawn, who was walking towards me.

"Keith and Natalie are here," Shawn began as we closed to talking distance. "Keith is right over there playing blackjack and I don't know where Natalie went. Let's go over and see what their plans are today. How did you end up doing at poker?"

I funneled my venom into my story, as if I were the only man in Vegas who had lost money on a bad beat.

"The dumbasses cleaned me out. I was surrounded by people who didn't know how to play, and they kept winning hands they had no business being in. The very last hand, this guy won with two pair, a pair of threes and sixes. It was such shit. I already blew through most of today's money, too. I think I'm going to need to take a break and watch you guys play some before I play anymore, or I'm not going to have anything left for tomorrow."

Shawn suffered through the story sympathetically, since he probably thought we would all have a couple of these to tell by the end of the trip, and believed I would have to listen to his complaints at a later time. We eventually reached Keith, who was getting up from his table.

"'Sup guys? It's been a while, Neil," Keith said, as he rose from his seat and shook my hand. "You finished losing at poker, or do you want to find a table where I can take your money?"

"I wouldn't mind giving you my money as much as I did losing it to the dumbasses at the last table. Right now I am going to sit a few out, but maybe in a little bit. Where's Natalie?"

"She's playing the slots, but she'll be back in a few minutes. I had some luck with Craps the last time I was here, so that is the next stop."

I tagged along with them to the Craps table and watched them play, but I couldn't figure out what was going on. Natalie found us a half hour later, and she was carrying a bucket of change. She had hit on a couple of desired combinations while in front of the demonstrative machine, and she had the all-that-glitters to prove it. I hadn't seen her since their wedding, and we exchanged a friendly hello hug before returning our eyes to the action.

I itched to play again, but remembered how low my funds were, and I bought drinks as I continued to watch a game I didn't understand. Even though I didn't understand the rules, I could tell Keith and Shawn were not doing particularly well, and they were soon ready to move on.

Since Shawn wanted to play Blackjack, we headed to a nearby table. It was late afternoon, so the tables were sparsely populated, and the minimum bets were low. I watched him play for a few minutes and tried to re-familiarize myself with the strategy of the game, like when one should hit and when one should stay. Finally, I decided to join him. Though Blackjack wasn't my game of choice, the bets were small enough that I could play cheaply and justify my losses with the free drinks.

The game suited my tastes perfectly. If you asked the dealer what to do, he or she would tell you what the conventional wisdom was in that particular situation. Multiple people could win. Gin and tonic in hand, I embarked on my career as a blackjack player.

Initially, Shawn and I were doing okay but not spectacularly well. Still, we were doing well enough that we knew we would be drunk before we lost our money. This was a godsend for me, since I had withdrawn another $200 and there wasn't anything left for the evening, and not much more budgeted for the trip. But I was, without even realizing it, very slowly accumulating some winnings.

It was probably on the third gin and tonic at the table that I entered into a Guy Richie movie. Everything around me moved as if it was in fast forward and I sat at the table with a single-minded focus. I believed that mine was a system of unrivaled genius grounded in simplicity. I quit betting my cards. I calculated that the dealer generally busted about once every three times. So I bet the minimum, and if the dealer hadn't busted in three hands, I threw back the remnants of my gin and tonic and bet the maximum I could bet.

With every win, I moved a few chips into a reserve pile I would no longer touch, to ensure that I ended the evening ahead. Each win was systematically divided. Part went into reserves, one or two chips went to the dealer, another made it onto the cocktail waitress's tray to ensure she kept returning with more fuel, and the remaining chips restocked my ammunition.

Shawn got bored and left the table to find something else to do. I hardly even noticed. My stacks of chips kept growing, and the dealer kept asking me to color up. I hadn't seen sobriety in hours when Shawn returned with Keith to check on me. On the table in front of me rested piles of different colored chips, showing how successful I had been. My proclamation was not as easily intelligible, and they looked on, laughing, as I sat swaying on my stool and kept winning, before they finally moved on to new sources of entertainment. The minimum bet rose, but I was grandfathered in at the lower rate, and my success came at a cheaper price than it did for the other people who came and left. My dealer's vocal range extended from bass to alto, and his physique morphed so many times that a police sketch artist would have drawn a Picasso.

Shawn stopped by the table to let me know that he was done for the night and to remind me of the room number. A few hours later, I lost two big hands, and it was time for bed. I tossed the dealer another $20 chip, and a woman came by and helped me take my chips to the front to cash them out. I had turned $200 into over $2500. I put the money in a safe at the hotel, and then I looked at my watch. It was two a.m. I had paid for my flight, my hotel room, and my drinks and still made some money.

The rest of the weekend was a drunken blur devoid of any memories. I would lose about $800 of that money over the next day, at the tables, I suppose, but I had no idea how. I ate a buffet breakfast replete with mimosas, and I never again flirted with sobriety. My friends went to Cirque Du Soleil. I played cards and drank. The world flew by, and I lived comfortably in my intoxicated cocoon. I loved Vegas.

{chapter 31}

To be more precise, I loved the escape of Vegas. But reality still awaited me in Atlanta, and there were countless problems with it. Some of those suddenly occurred to me as the plane descended. My resume had enormous holes in it. My memory flirted with being useful but abandoned me randomly, guaranteeing I could not depend on it. I had friends in Atlanta, but they had grueling jobs that occupied their time, income streams to fund their hobbies, and significant others with whom they planned their lives. Our friendships were founded while we were on equal footing, but that was no longer the case. Even before I'd left Vegas, I had been emailing them to set up times for drinks or movies or dinners during the week, but they had always politely declined, since they were busy with work or had plans with others already in place.

I continued ticking through the problems as we lost altitude. I looked athletic, but my balance was still so prone to disappearing that standing felt like a temporary state at best. The wave of random illnesses that had plagued me over the last two years had slowed, but I knew these health problems, or "tax on being alive" as I used to call them, lurked in the shadows. I was single, insecure, whiney, depressed, embarrassingly self-absorbed, unemployed, and without a single discernable job skill. There was a lot of reality to embrace as the wheels finally touched down in Atlanta. The future looked bleak, further stoking my fatalism. I knew there were a lot of twos in my rating future.

My big dreams had never died quick deaths—I remained convinced of the near-certainty of my professional athletic career until age seventeen. This particular instance was no exception. I was surrounded not only by warning signs that I could not resume the life to which I had once felt destined but by affirmative evidence that even what I considered mediocrity was a bit too ambitious. I wasn't in a rush to turn around and face what I knew was approaching. So I didn't. I had become too good at escaping. Instead, I bought gifts with my Vegas winnings and went home for Christmas.

"Colin may be coming to Atlanta," Mom informed me my first morning home, with my brother silently sitting right next to me at the kitchen table in Aiken.

"I applied, but I haven't even had my interview yet," Colin explained before returning to his cereal.

Mom had mentioned this possibility over the phone before. He was considering an internship with the Centers for Disease Control in Atlanta. It was one of the most prestigious internships you could get while still in medical school. The competition for the position was fierce, but he had applied anyway. For a lot of people, this meant little other than beginning a long process that could end in one of two ways. Colin had never been one of these people in Mom's eyes, or for that matter, in mine either. My brother was coming to Atlanta. This would be confirmed by May.

We wound down the festivities, and Colin headed back to Charleston. My Christmas haul was, as usual, bountiful, and Mom also packed me off to Atlanta with a cooler full of food and a head full of her stock advice.

"Be disciplined, Neil. Meet with your career counselor, explore all of your options, and spend this time figuring out your next steps. You need to stay on top of this. There are jobs out there that you would like. You need to keep looking. Don't get discouraged. You are bright, and employers are looking for young people like you. Make sure you get your resume out there. Don't doubt yourself just because those two jobs didn't work out. And don't lead with your wreck. It isn't something your employer needs to know."

The great thing about Mom's talks was that they were positive and they always stuck with me. No matter how little factual basis lay behind her conclusions, I managed to believe what she told me. I was charming, smart, funny, and athletic. She would defend this concept to the death because I was her son.

But she hadn't seen these failures from the ground floor. The people around me on a daily basis knew my struggles firsthand, and they knew the truth. Chad dropped hints, always couched in terms of "when I worked with you," but I wasn't going to face reality until someone got in my face and yelled it.

My friends weren't the people best suited for this job. I was going to resent the messenger. And even after I felt like I had lost so much, I still had "maybe," that unattainable flirt and purveyor of false hope. Maybe I would magically heal. Maybe everything would soon get better. My friends didn't want to be the dream killers, to tell me that my time in the dream world was up, especially when no one—not doctors, not even neurologists—could predict my recovery trajectory with any certainty. Everyone was forced to sit silently and watch me flail.

Mom was certainly not to be the provider of this elusive truth that I wouldn't embrace. She wasn't even armed with the facts. She was removed from the action and only heard about the problems over the phone and, accustomed to my doom-and-gloom outlook, assumed it was always another exaggeration. She, like me, might have known but not wanted to.

I sped back toward the angry snarl of reality, unprepared for the harshness of its delivery. For two and a half hours, as interstate signs passed, I talked myself into believing a dream scenario that I suspected was false. By the time I arrived in Atlanta, I had ideas about how to tweak my resume, so I sat down in front of my computer to make it perfect. Then I set to work with the flashcards and books Wendy had given me. I needed a job, and using the tools at my disposal, it was only a matter of time before I would find it.

There was still too much uncertainty in this fight, so the next day, I created a schedule. Each hour of every day during the week was planned. My meals, whether breakfast or lunch, were opportunities for informational interviews with people whose contact information I had obtained through my friends and acquaintances and who worked in fields that interested me. I scheduled weekly workouts with my trainer and noted the number of hours I would train each day on my own on my calendar. I made time to explore interesting subjects, during which I planned to read The Economist to learn about the world around me while improving my vocabulary, or I would read books that might be helpful for business conversations, such as The Tipping Point.

I specified in my calendar exactly when my weekly meetings with Wendy were scheduled and how long I would work on the career books she provided to determine the specific careers I should apply for. I blocked off large periods of time to research companies and submit resumes for jobs outside of law for which I thought I would qualify.

I even allocated time for introspection, assuming this was an activity separate from my other daily activities. I liberally set aside two to three hours a week for the necessary exploration of self, whether it consisted of Internet research into brain injuries so I could create workable compensation strategies, emailing old friends from law school to cement my connections with people holding essential missing knowledge, or going to the head injury support group once a month, where someone might have "the answers." The structured world I built would prevent laziness. In a universe of uncertainty, my system would eliminate the risk of failure. Like Vegas, I had an infallible system that, if followed, would guarantee my success.

Every day I obeyed it, and during our meetings, I listened to Wendy's suggestions and tried to incorporate them into my plan. I met with anyone who would meet with me. With the nuances Wendy suggested and those that my my experiences were providing, the system was evolving to become a perfect machine.

The messenger who first delivered damnation was silent. The resumes weren't even getting nibbles. I was casting electronic documents into the blackness with no idea why the booming voice beckoning me to the Promised Land would not ring out. I was out of time for patience. I didn't have months to wait for everything to fall into place, especially knowing how unlikely such an occurrence had been in the past. Money was evaporating too quickly. Frustration was fast becoming the dominant emotion once again. After a few weeks, my system wasn't working, and I declared it a failure. There was too much uncertainty for this farce to continue.

Hopelessness is a relative term, and in its relativity, excuses are born. What appears hopeless to some looks fortuitous to others, and this undoubtedly was the case in my situation. Every day someone had promised me tomorrow would be better, even while I lay tied to a hospital bed. This incarnation of hopelessness was a result of knowing for months that today's promise was a lie. The hard work of recovery was supposed to be completed in the hospital, and I was to coast into my overly-idealized view of the future; too many months of persistent problems made tomorrow, with its unconquerable obstacles, worse than today. My new visions were of an apocalyptic future, with its burned-out buildings lining a deserted road, desolate and devoid of promise, replacing the previously-imagined manicured street I intended to call home. The stunning wife who had once waved to me from the porch of my McMansion in the fantastical future no longer appeared. The world I found myself looking into wasn't right. This was not my beautiful house. It was too much for me to stomach.

That's what hopeless was to me: a moment when I knew I could not guide my future into the dock I had built of expectations at age twenty-four. I had dealt with the present decently well—other than those moments of terror, even my first memories of lying in my hospital bed had been hopeful, my mind echoing the pronouncements of a full recovery that Mom made on a daily basis. But I suddenly knew the future reward toward which I had been diligently working would never be delivered. I was now defined by the absence of a career. I was a sprinter by nature, and my efforts, as slight as they might appear to most, seemed worthy of at least some feedback, yet I received none.

I didn't know what else to do to at least elicit some response. If I were told that my resume clearly painted me as incompetent and showed that I would make a horrible employee, I would find a way to convincingly extol my virtues and potential employers would stop seeing only the flaws. But to these companies, who held in their hands a document that purported to reveal my business background, my summarized identity wasn't even worthy of a response. I had grown to expect rejection, but corporate ambivalence regarding my future was something I could not handle.

"Don't give up so easily. It has barely been a month," Mom reminded me during one evening's phone conversation.

It had been longer. It had been over two years. This particular instance did not stand alone. It joined the "canon of no" that all of my experiences left me to reference.

But maybe it was me choosing to focus only on these. There were many good times that had occurred as frequently as, if not more than, the bad. I had enjoyed beers with my friends in Atlanta, hearty Thanksgiving dinners, and trips to visit friends in other cities. And I had once amazed everyone with my rapid recovery. My failure had often been predicted in places where I then succeeded.

I knew it was way too early to give up, but I was tired. I had fought this battle for two years. It was time to retreat. The collapse that followed was pathetically self-destructive but otherwise muted to everyone else. I played the game during the day.

"There is nothing to see here, so keep moving," my actions informed anyone interested enough to consider pausing for a closer look. I went to my appointments, I made my calls, and I assured Mom I was making progress. But in the evenings, I lifted the bottle of escape, and I welcomed self-destruction with a passion with which I had not embraced life in ages. Unlike Vegas, my goals during this session were wholly different; there was no fun to be had and certainly no system to put into place. I wanted it to be done, but in the passive way of a boy too unsure to make a "yes" or "no" decision about a subject he'd been considering for two years. I still made sure to play my part when anyone might be looking, in case I was making the wrong decision. I was non-committal even as I quietly quit.

The illusion ended by five every day that week, and my mind forgot to retain information as I continued my evening drive toward oblivion. Intermittently, I sobered up enough to show up for a friend's party at a nearby bar, but by the time I returned, I was blind drunk. And so it went.

For five days, I did little to ensure my survival, but I never really quit. I only sporadically remembered to eat, but I still left my afternoons open for productive activities, and I only overbooked my evenings with surrender. It wasn't a cry for help, because no one was around to observe it. It was simply another failed attempt to deal with the unknowable.

That final day, six days after I had begun this trip, I woke and felt a kind of fear like nothing I had ever experienced. My memory—all but one image—had left, but there was other carnage too, and my mind could not explain the panic. Unlike previous post-wreck experiences, I was not sifting through shards of memories, hoping to piece it back together. There was nothing more than a single picture. But something had happened.

I was missing my ATM card, and I called the bank to cancell it. My online account statement showed that I had withdrawn $120 that I didn't remember taking out, then someone had withdrawn $380, the maximum amount allowed, later that night when I thought I was in bed. Someone had also used my debit card to buy a full tank of gas. I was trying to figure out my evening and my finances with a hangover five days in the making when I realized I might never know what happened, and though part of me was relieved by that, I was mostly terrified.

Even without any sensory data from the night, I had an unshakeable feeling I had done something bad, and I knew without knowing that there had been a woman whose interests were purely monetary. I couldn't explain why. I had one image, the inside of a car from the passenger seat as the car moved along, and I had no idea why I would have been in a car, much less who the driver was. None of this made sense. I stood in the shower scrubbing until my skin was raw, my pulse racing in panic.

There were countless possibilities for what had happened, and none of them were good. With the scorching hot water running off me, the bar of soap melting down as I ran it vigorously across the visible ribs on my sides, I considered possible explanations for why I felt such terror, for why I was missing so much money. I didn't dwell in the rational for too long before I jumped into Hollywood horrors.

I felt certain I had not driven, since my first order of business had been to check on my car, and it was parked where I left it the previous afternoon. It didn't appear that I had killed anyone, since the news was not reporting an incident of any kind in the area from that night. This wasn't even a plausible explanation. It explained only my racing pulse and the increased feeling of impending doom. But someone had taken out that money, and I knew it wasn't me, and for this, I had no explanation. And I knew there had been a woman. That was all I knew.

The water never cooled, but after fifteen minutes, I turned it off and toweled myself dry. Once I was in my car, I immediately headed to the nearby doc-in-the-box to get a full battery of tests, including a blood test. I needed him to tell me it was going to be okay.

"The blood test could give a false negative for a while," the doctor instead informed me. "If you're concerned about something that happened last night, blood tests will probably not show anything yet."

I knew it was a waste of time and a waste of money, but I had them do the tests anyway. What a buffoon. I was too scared to think it through. The list of things I would never fully know about the prior evening was alarming even to someone as accustomed to memory loss as I, and the only thing I knew for certain was that I wanted to be alive. The binge had ended on day six, and though the testing would continue for the next year, I was finally attached to my existence with enough conviction that I did not plan on abandoning it.

{chapter 32}

The shame, which had once simply been a product of failure, transformed into something far more overwhelming when it was grounded in one event, completely unintelligible as it was, as opposed to two years of inadequate efforts. Every blackout experience—and due to my brain's inability to handle alcohol competently, there were many—raised with it the possibility of an ominous event missing from my memory, and I revisited them one at a time. I was missing much of my Vegas memory and I couldn't accurately explain what happened to some of the money I had won. What had happened there? Or was it all in my head, a new made-up horror story with which I could torture myself?

It felt too real to be completely psychosomatic, but so had my previous jaw pain. I began the flagellation without any conviction, hoping my guilt would soon begin to dissipate. I eschewed fun, as if it were something I was prone to engaging in too regularly. I resumed my regimented schedule, since it brought me peace of mind. And I redoubled my efforts to become involved in charitable causes, whether I was tutoring underprivileged kids or working with the brain injury charity, mostly because I enjoyed feeling like my existence benefitted someone else, and I wanted to get away from my unemployed position, where I strongly disliked my boss.

The following week, I was in my car, about to go into my Shepherd Center Junior Committee meeting to continue my charitable penance, when my phone rang. It was Alicia, which usually meant the conversation would last for the duration of her drive to her next destination, keeping it under five minutes. Since I was about ten minutes early, I picked it up.

"Heeeaay," she greeted me in the child-like, high-pitched Southern drawl that made her sound friendly and non-threatening. "How's everything going?"

She must be going across town, I thought, and I didn't have too much spare time.

"Everything is going pretty well. I'm about to head into a volunteer meeting. Can I call you back tonight?"

"Sure. I wanted to see what you were doing this weekend, make sure you're still free."

"I don't have any plans." I knew that I wouldn't be having fun. I could feel the welts.

"I have a wedding in Huntsville, and I don't have a date, so I was wondering if maybe I could drive to Atlanta, pick you up, and we could go together. The reception is being held at the NASA space center, so it should be fun."

"I could probably do that. I'll just need to check my calendar when I get home tonight."

"Great! Give me a call tonight, then. This would be a huge help. It's Jerry and Heather's wedding, you know, the couple who threw the Halloween party. I've dated a couple of the groomsmen, so I can't go to this thing by myself."

"All right, I am pretty sure I can go with you, but I'll need to confirm it tonight. I need to go in now, but I'll call you later."

I hung up and walked inside to join the group of civic-minded people intent on helping injured individuals through fundraising.

That Friday, I was riding shotgun in the Jeep that Alicia piloted, headed to Alabama.

"Do you remember them from the costume party where I went as Daisy Duke?" she asked.

"Yes, they both seemed nice. I didn't get a chance to talk to them much, but I don't think I'll run into them other than to say hey a couple of times this weekend."

"I'll introduce you to some of the people I know tonight at the rehearsal dinner," she said. "This is going to be lots of fun."

I would meet loads of people that evening at the rehearsal dinner. I recognized a few of them from the party. I remembered no names.

The wedding the next day went smoothly, at least to my untrained eye, like weddings are supposed to go, and we headed back to the space center for the reception. Everyone was in good spirits, the anticipation of a promising future permeating even the most disillusioned people's temperaments. Unbridled optimism was always my favorite part of weddings, and seeing the genuine looks of happiness on the faces of the bride and groom as they took their seats at the front and looked out on the adoring throng of well-wishers made me believe, if only for a few minutes, that everything worked out in the end.

My second favorite part of weddings was the bar, though tonight I visited it with some degree of reserve, choosing beer over its fiercer cousin liquor, and piling my plate high with the incredible food provided to the guests to cushion its blow. Alicia and I found our seats, and I set to work demolishing the course in front of me. Conscious that people actually came to weddings to socialize, not simply mooch free food and drinks, I looked up in search of someone with whom I could engage in a meaningful discussion about their career or the absence of mine. A woman named Donna showed a willingness to participate with me in such a conversation.

"I live in New York City. I'm a television producer for one of the networks."

The food was suddenly not as interesting, and I applied some additional social lubricant to the situation. Alicia was engaging the object of my interest's date in a similar discussion. He was a hand surgeon. I knew I didn't fit in but, for once, I didn't care.

Still haunted by my recent past, I consumed the beers with some reserve as I listened to Donna detail a world I had never even thought to dream about. She was behind the lens and, as we talked, I began to understand more about her role. She tracked down leads, interviewed alleged killers to get their stories, and tried to use all of her resources to offer viewers insight into the unseemly side of human nature in a manner that the American public could casually digest.

When it came time for me to reveal my life happenings, I delivered my story with such conviction that the Academy would have been proud. I spoke not of my recent past, analogous to the story she had just finished delivering, but the only one I knew to tell, the story of why I wasn't. I had rehearsed these lines for so long that they were second nature, but I altered my focus a bit this time. I concentrated not on the end result, the brain injury, but on the horrors of the incident itself to explain precisely why my memory still lay in that hospital bed even when I had long since departed, borrowing from the police report and hospital intake sheets I had read to recount specific details of the accident.

After hearing about the seriousness of the wreck, she could understand why the recovery had taken so long. It generally wasn't my mind that was the problem. She could hear the vocabulary words rolling off my tongue. It wasn't the emotional instability that wracked me on a daily basis. Tears never rolled down my cheek, so she remained unaware of this issue. It was my memory, and since everything else was beginning to return, she could see that this would eventually come back, too. It was simply a matter of time.

She nodded empathetically. She listened to sob-stories for a living, and her non-verbal cues promised compassion.

I wasn't the only one drinking, and after about two hours of small talk and some dancing, the conversation took a rather blunt turn.

"I have really enjoyed talking with you. Would you like to step out into the hall? I want to kiss and see if we have chemistry."

Only at a wedding, after an evening of drinking, would this seem like a logical request, but that night, it made sense. I took another sip of my beer and got up from the empty table to join her in the hall, thinking about precisely how I would approach this, movie kisses flashing through my head. I had one chance to get this right. I analyzed all the different options in my head.

The next morning, as I headed back to my room before breakfast after a sleepover, I was happy. The specific guilt I had so recently harbored, a guilt that had once threatened to swallow me, would be allowed visiting privileges, but it was no longer the central tenant in my life. Donna's date, Ryan, emerged from my room at the same time I made it back. I jumped into the shower and changed into traveling clothes, and while I packed my other clothes, I listened to Alicia debate the pros and cons of her evening companion. By the time we made it down for breakfast before we hit the road, the story had spread among a few of Alicia's friends.

"Date swap, huh?" one of Alicia's friends said, as we approached a table with our plate of food.

I nervously laughed and averted my eyes sheepishly.

Donna and Ryan sat with us a few minutes later, and I spent the meal chatting with her.

"I was going to ride back with Ryan, but he needs to get back earlier than I do. My flight out isn't until later. I could ride back with you guys, if you could take me to the airport."

And with that, we had another passenger. Donna and I took the back seat while Alicia chauffeured us to Atlanta. I'm not sure how I justified this as socially acceptable behavior, but we did keep Alicia included in our conversation. Once we got back to Atlanta, we grabbed an early dinner at Rio Grande, a

Mexican place close to my house, where we sat and laughed about the weekend's events.

I came to learn two things, which were not completely clear to me during the previous evening. Donna was my senior by a few years, and she was Jewish. Since I was not particularly religious, nor was I offended by the idea of seeing someone older than me, this did not seem to be an obstacle, and we continued to hang out at my apartment even when Alicia had to leave to finish her trip back to Columbia. Eventually, I took Donna to the airport, and we said goodbye as she made her way to the security line that guarded her terminal.

As I watched her pass through the gate and move toward her terminal, I realized I possibly had the beginnings of a long distance relationship with someone new. I was confused by the fact that she could still look at me and see something appealing, even after she had learned that there was so much wrong, but I was thankful. I thought there might come a day when I could burden her with my insecurities and talk through my problems with her to arrive at better solutions, once everything between us stabilized. She seemed willing to join me on my confusing journey. I didn't feel quite as alone anymore. I had found a woman who would serve both as a confidante and a new distraction from the chaos.

{chapter 33}

My life remained schizophrenic. There were no pauses allowing for continuity. Though my personal life was suddenly showing promise, nothing else was. I received frequent calls and emails from Donna, and even visits every couple of weekends. Potential employers weren't nearly so interested. The dream of restoration to my legal throne was dead. At last, with no further options available, I began to acknowledge what Wendy was saying. Networking was the key. I had to figure out what job I wanted, and then, using my resources, learn about the job and how to acquire such a position.

My quest for professional self began again, and, this time, I finally understood. I needed to embrace the personal connections made during the course of my life while not binding myself to the life paths that no longer suited my new identity. The old me, with his childish materialism and immature view of success, would no longer hinder my progress, but I could use him. I had met people along the way who liked me, or at least didn't have a physical aversion to my presence. These people were the key. They would provide information while I searched for my own answers. I made a list of anyone who potentially could serve as a business contact and then began looking for the job that might make me happy.

I tutored underprivileged children once a week and loved the time I spent with them. They laughed as they learned, and when I sent them home with the addition and multiplication flashcards I had made with blank note cards and a Sharpie, they guarded them as though my gift was priceless. Learning was not yet a chore, and I felt revitalized around them during that hour once a week.

I volunteered at park clean-ups, and my fellow volunteers chatted while working alongside me, happy to be there. Any job posted on the Hands on Atlanta website that I felt comfortable trying, I signed up for and met people of various backgrounds who, at the very least, portrayed happy people as convincingly as skilled actors during our limited time together. It occurred to me that I was seeing these people at their best, but when I thought back to how miserable my former colleagues had been at work, I wondered if their jobs had reduced even their free time to a countdown to dread. These new people did not operate in such a manner, and I could borrow their optimism.

The old self I had audibly forsaken did not relinquish control permanently, and part of me still viewed every moment outside the business universe I once occupied as wasted time. I was burning through my savings rapidly even as I slashed expenses, and I was terrified of the day when there was no remaining fuel for my life. Like most people who find themselves unemployed, I couldn't force myself to simply enjoy my time away and learn new lessons while I was planning for my next opportunity. Instead, I continued to dump resume after resume into the stream of commerce, praying that someone would offer me a job, blind to what I was then witnessing.

I thought there must be someone willing to hire me, and this hope was what dominated every thought outside my forays into volunteerism. Every day without interest was another reminder of the situation's bleakness. Once a month, I wrote the $460 check to my old employer to keep my health insurance after it became clear that I was simply uninsurable outside of COBRA. I paid my rent, and to conserve my finite funds, I stopped leaving my apartment except on official business. The market's gains erased many of my withdrawals, but I knew this could not go on forever. I needed a source of income.

Within three months, I stopped looking for what I wanted and resumed looking for what I could get. At one of my

informational interviews with a friend of a friend, my guest
discussed consulting work with me. She felt that my law degree
could still be useful to me in a consulting position, if that was
what I was looking for. She explained her daily routine with
enough specificity that I could talk myself into being readily
qualified for such a job, despite not fully understanding what
she had described.

I had spent my recent past creating procedures that ensured
efficiencies in my own life; surely I could talk someone into
offering me a position doing the same thing on a larger scale. I
didn't have a business degree, like most of their candidates did,
but I had a work finance background, law school experience that
taught linear thinking patterns and problem solving, and I was
pretty sure my mind would work this time around. This was the
job I was qualified for today, so it was what I was looking for.

As I began the application process and saw all of the blanks,
the fit no longer seemed as perfect. I hadn't attended business
school, and all the applications seemed to assume that I had.
At this point, I didn't have any professors who remembered me.
The forms asked for a recommendation from my last employer.
I'd willingly provide the name, but I hardly expected a reference,
and this was what the forms requested. Without another easy
option, I fell on the mercy of the Court.

"Cole Hyde," the cheerful voice answered.

"Hello, this is Neil Ligon, may I speak with Alan?"

"One moment, please."

After a lengthy pause, but before my will had collapsed, he
picked up.

"Alan speaking."

"Hi Alan, it is Neil."

"Neil, what can I do for you?"

His tone wasn't brusque; it was friendly enough. I could do
this. Using the machine gun cadence that marked my tenure at

his firm, I launched into my spiel before nerves rendered me mute.

"You mentioned in our final correspondence that you considered the fact that I did not work out at your firm as a personal failure. I wanted to clarify something. You were not in any way to blame. I had a car accident right after I took the bar that I almost died in. My memory still didn't work properly, and I couldn't retain what you were teaching me. I have decided to leave the field of law and go into consulting, and I wanted to let you know that some of these companies may contact you. I didn't want you to be surprised, and I wanted you to understand my situation when they asked about my time at the firm."

A three-beat of silence offered promise. I had finally perfected the telling of the story. Water under the bridge, he would say. Your story is courageous. What an impressive tale. I would have never known. That must have been hard on your mother. You should become a motivational speaker with such a heart-wrenching story. He did not read his lines.

"Were you fired from Irwin Myers?" he asked instead.

"No, but they put me on probation," I answered quickly. The ad-libbing made me nervous. I needed to know where this was going. He continued to press.

"Were you going to be fired?"

"Once they put me on probation, I started looking for jobs," I shakily explained, while I silently begged him to stop. "At the end of that time, I would have probably been given an extra couple of weeks to find a job before they fired me."

"Did the head-hunter you used know about this?" he persisted.

"No, I didn't tell anyone." Except my softball team. And anyone around me after four beers. And a couple of my friends.

"I knew something was wrong. Even during the probationary period, I knew something was wrong, but I thought you were nervous, and so we kept you on. I don't know what I would have done in your position, but you lied to me," he practically yelled into the phone. "That money could have paid for a semester of my son's tuition at UGA. Are you going to tell these firms about your wreck?"

The tone was hostile and the volume loud. I hadn't conveyed the story properly. Didn't he understand? I was following doctors' orders. It wasn't my fault. I was trying to survive… without giving up my lifestyle…at his expense. Maybe I didn't understand. It was too late to turn back. I hoped the line would go dead. A lightning strike could take down a pole and terminate the call. It was sunny outside.

"No, I'm not going to tell them. I think my memory is coming back. Everyone tells me it is getting better. I think I can do the work now." Reading The Economist, Fortune and Time Magazine, the on-line Cal Berkley economics lectures, the flashcards with vocabulary words that were beginning to stick, all the workouts—they had to mean something. I was healing. I would soon be whole. I just needed another chance. Again.

"You are lying to a new group of people. I can't discuss your work while you were here, but this conversation is outside of that scope. I can share what we talked about today. I do not have anything more to say to you."

The line went dead. I jumped up and ran to the bathroom, where my body reflexively heaved the churning stomach acid halfway up my throat before it returned to its home and left me to stare at my distorted reflection in the empty toilet bowl. Everything he had said was true, at least from his perspective. My resume required clarification, and if I didn't explain this, I was in many ways lying about the past. In this instance, I couldn't look out for myself and someone else simultaneously. Was it my job too? He seemed to think it was, and he had persuaded me.

There wasn't a handbook for how to handle job interviews when you could effectively hide your handicaps and your past employers could not disclose what they knew. I was making it up as I went. I had solicited input from medical professionals and reintegration specialists, but they weren't employing me. They didn't understand the complexity of the jobs for which I was applying.

I returned to my desk and typed a quick email to him admitting my errors in judgment, a belated mea culpa, as if this would solve the problems. It was now me against the world. Everyone else got to look out for themselves, inside the bounds of legality, and I had to figure out how to protect myself while living my life at the discretion of everyone else.

"What you see is a lie," I was to announce as I walked into every job interview. "I do not want you to get confused. I want you to understand exactly why you shouldn't hire me. I had a horrible wreck, and I have a brain injury. I don't know what all of my limitations are. No one can tell me what they are, but there are many of them. Thus, the first part of my resume showing my school successes isn't accurate. You should start and stop at the Employment Experience section, except I gained those positions by deception, and once they learned the truth, they were going to fire me, so ignore any prestige which these jobs might convey. Please focus on the firings. Assume I am useless. I will soon."

"I am only qualified for manual labor jobs," I hurt into the phone. It was another lie. My disappearing balance rendered me useless for such a position. I was a dishwasher for life.

I ignored Mom's response, because it didn't matter. This was simply another pity party, and I needed a witness for the collapse. If someone could document it, this one could count. It could be put toward my sentence for all the mistakes I had made, all the immoral things I had ever done, all the people I had hurt. I needed to be released early for good behavior, or at least read my sentence. This could not extend into perpetuity.

My resume, dripping with misleading statements, finally contained enough truth to punish, and it bore the appropriate fruit with the apathy it elicited from others. I had worked for two employers in two years, the second of which lasted less than a year. There weren't any interviews on the horizon. The deception was to end, since it was no longer an option. The phone never rang, there were no emails in my inbox, and though I check it diligently, I found that my spam filter only kept out offers to fix potential physical inadequacies, not offers of employment. I deactivated my Georgia Bar membership. It was time to fold up shop and run. Again. I packed my bags for New York. I had a woman to visit.

{chapter 34}

She was an active participant in my self-discovery, even while she was living in New York, so it seemed odd to escape reality by traveling to the epicenter of my search for it. She had sent me articles and told me stories of people overcoming the problems I struggled with on a daily basis. She didn't just ignore that I was unemployed, she announced in the presence of others that it was a temporary problem that I would soon overcome. She introduced me over email and talked about me with her friends. My shame was not hers. She had not seen the problems every day. She hadn't heard the silence responding to my job entreaties. I was broken, but the breaks didn't look too bad, because I was new.

I could run away to this, so I made the arrangements. We planned all of the details. There was a birthday dinner for two of her friends. One of the people having a birthday was a woman who worked as a television news producer. Donna knew her from an earlier job, and the woman's husband was a National Geographic photographer. The following day we would depart for another close friend's house, located in the Pennsylvania countryside. This friend was a freelance anchor for various national news programs, and her friend's husband was a successful venture capitalist. Donna had forwarded his photo to me via email—in it he was standing with presidential candidate Senator Barack Obama. We would come back Monday to catch a Jon Stewart show, where one of her friends worked as a writer. The escape from my reality could not have been more complete.

My visit to New York was hardly intended to mirror her frequent visits to Atlanta, where I had simply introduced her to my friends and visited local sports bars, but we knew there were differences between the two of us, measurable both numerically and by way of affiliation, and she had never pointed these things out. I was unemployed and pathetic, but she willingly buoyed my faltering confidence while aiding my development. The timing of my winter visit to New York would be perfect. I could see her world and hide in it. Her friends would accept me as a courtesy to Donna—not as an equal, of course, but as a tolerable interloper. Everything would be okay once I got there. The intervening cause arrived first.

"It's snowing here. Check your flight status. It isn't snowing hard," her email informed me.

The snow continued to fall harder, and her correspondence, spread out over the next few hours, reflected the growing unlikelihood that this trip would occur.

"I'm still on hold. I hope you can get a flight in, maybe something tomorrow morning."

"See if Newark gives you a better chance of getting in."

"They are only cancelling flights to NYC. You can fly to Philly and take an hour train ride to NYC."

"We tried."

The promise of escape evaporated. I was left behind. It wasn't her fault, nor was it mine. Sometimes things went this way. It wasn't the end of the world. No one had died. It was just a cancelled flight. I'd see her when she was in Atlanta for work in less than a month. It was finally time to face reality.

I returned to the bleakness of my glowing computer screen. My resume looked as hideous as it had the day before. This time I didn't go for a beer to help me wash down what I was taking in. I instead began to stare it down, to sculpt it in my mind into the object of beauty it was supposed to be. I would eliminate the precise dates to disguise how short my tenure at the other positions had been. I measured failures in generality; successes I illustrated with precision. I noticed with pride how the Extracurricular category was growing more populated. There was hope in those tutoring sessions. I saved the document to the desktop and opened my browser to begin my Macro Economics lecture.

{chapter 35}

Sitting in my living room, I was able to grab the phone next to me by the second ring, and a verbal flurry answered my "hello."

"How's it going? Quick question: Mark Burress—do you remember him? He was my ex-boyfriend from Tulane—graduated and doesn't have a job. Do you think it would be insulting if I forwarded this job opening to him? It's just a document review job, but the pay is decent. It would be something to put on his resume for now. What do you think?"

It was Jill, my friend in Atlanta from the Tulane Law Review. Jill was a fast talker. When I had seen her number, I anticipated a discussion of evening plans, and her opening's unexpected subject had left me struggling to find a response. Though her rapid beginning hadn't allowed much time to think, I did so in the moments that followed, buying time with verbal filler.

"Hey, Jill. Um…."

My mind churned while my mouth whirred. My email inbox still sat empty and my phone had been relegated exclusively to my incoming personal calls. The dollar amount in my bank account grew smaller every day. I had no idea whether Mark would find this job offer insulting. I knew that I would give a kidney for a job interview, and this was the closest I had gotten in four months.

I treaded carefully. No one wanted the friend who didn't understand his place. I had failed at two jobs already. Why would someone want their name affiliated with my work performance? What made me think I could do this one? Desperation was the catalyst for the words that followed. I needed to exhaust all my options before I started washing dishes. My voice finally caught.

"I don't know about Mark, but that sounds like something I would be interested in."

I sounded pathetic. I felt my face flush with blood, and I was thankful that she could not witness this visual display. She changed gears with the speed of the successful.

"Oh, I didn't think about you, since you said you were looking to get out of law. I think it would be a great fit. I think their hours are pretty reasonable. And I don't know a lot of the people over there, but Dennis is super nice. If you're interested, shoot me your resume."

I wasn't convinced. She was just being nice. I wouldn't be able to do the work. My resume was dishonest. There were too many problems. Resignation to an inescapable fate was the noble thing to do. No one else would get hurt.

But I knew this position would only be temporary. How much damage could I cause in such a short time? I continued with my inquiries.

"Do you think I can do the work? Do you think I need to tell them about my wreck? I would only be there for a little while, but I don't want to have another run-in with a former employer. Do you think it would be okay?"

I needed her to sign off on it. I needed some guarantees.

"Neil, I am confident you could do the work. I think it's pretty straightforward. I don't see the need to tell them about the wreck. I think it will all be fine. Just send me your resume."

I remained doubtful, but without any other obvious options, and none of the less obvious options I was exploring paying any dividends, I didn't see that I had a choice. In the end, someone might yell at me again, but I could handle some mild verbal abuse. I probably wouldn't even get an interview, much less the job, anyway.

I reviewed my resume one final time. It was as mangled as it had been before. The lines were clean, the subheadings bolded and underlined, but they were merely inadequate sutures for a document still oozing incompetence. I double-checked the contact number it listed and prepared myself for the expected employer ambivalence.

Instead, after a lengthy enough pause that I had given up hope, I received an email to schedule a call. Within a week and a half, I had an in-person interview.

I arrived looking the part. The suit was nice, a relic of the days not too long before, when my apparent career path had led to purchases that I believed would be necessary in my future. The tie matched the pinstripe. I remembered my interviews, and I knew the procedures. Thankfully, there would be no opportunities to drink.

I practiced calm on the drive in. I needed to be honest about how long I planned to be there. I did not need to be honest about the wreck. I needed to be honest about my strengths. I did not know my weaknesses, so on that front, I would remain silent. I would smile the smile of the confident. I would avoid all attempts at humor. I would keep my answers short. I had no idea where I was going.

I glanced at my MapQuest directions, as if I couldn't see the building with the Star Wars strike fighter wings on its roof, but even as I arrived, I didn't know where to park. I felt the sweat running down my sides.

Stop panicking, I told myself. I needed to look like I had it together.

I parked the car and put on my coat to hide my sweat-stained shirt. The elevator let me out into the lobby, and I walked to the front desk as deliberately as my rapid pulse would allow.

Once I had my nametag, I was accepted, if only temporarily, and the gate allowed me in to the appropriate elevator bank, where I stepped on the latest arrival and began my ascent. I arrived at the designated floor a few minutes prior to the time I was expected, so I took a seat in the lobby with the graciousness that it was offered. I slipped the list of clients for whom I had worked at my earlier jobs out of my resume holder and input all of its data into the form I was completing, though my nervousness could be seen in my shaky handwriting. The only way to fix this problem was to relax.

Steady breathing began to take effect, and my jacket propounded the deceit set forth in the resume they already had. I was calm. I was well-educated. And with all the reading I was doing, I could appear articulate for twenty minutes.

They called me in, and I sat across the table from them as they looked over my resume. I already felt guilty by the time their eyes looked up. They introduced themselves as Leslie and Paul. I said hi, but otherwise kept silent. They didn't need to know.

Paul looked up first. "You know I went to Virginia for undergrad and Tulane for law school, too. And I started at Irwin Myers as well."

My "confident" smile disappeared. He was messing with me, but why? Did he know? Was this all a joke on me?

"Really?" I couldn't think of anything else to say. The sweating resumed.

"Yeah, I was two years ahead of you. But I was gone from Irwin Myers before you got there."

I finally sidestepped my panicking mind and followed the cues. "What group were you in?"

Names that I recognized filled the air. I had been there once. A weight was lifted and my squirming ceased as my smile reappeared. How fortuitous. I was finally getting the break to which I had so long believed I was entitled. I began to calm down as we discussed the old firm a bit before Leslie brought us back to the point.

"We are interviewing to fill an opening we have for a contract attorney. You would primarily be reviewing documents electronically. Your team leader would provide you with instructions for how you would handle the documents. Usually you would be determining if the documents are responsive to the subpoena. It requires precision and accuracy, but we have to work quickly as well. Does this sound like something you would be interested in?"

"Yes, that sounds perfect for right now," I answered her. "My experience at my last two positions taught me to have an eye for detail and to work efficiently. I am looking for something to hold me over while I transition out of law in the next couple of months, and this sounds like a great fit."

"We require a three-month commitment," she responded. "Will that be a problem?"

I would willingly promise her today in the hopes she could guarantee my tomorrows, so my answer was instantaneous. "I can promise three months."

From there, the questions that followed were cursory. She didn't fully explore why my previous jobs ended so rapidly. They both asked a few standard questions. The lie didn't grow too big.

"Thank you for your time, and we will be in touch after we finish interviewing and make our decisions."

I shook hands with both of them and left the room. After validating my parking with the receptionist, I took the elevator back down to ground level and returned my visitor badge to the security desk. There were so many screening checkpoints.

I would not work in that building for over a year. But a couple of days later, I received the call. Luck had found me a job, and I wasn't even concerned with what kind of job it was. I would resume my legal career with them at their other office, one that was a block away, above a daycare.

{chapter 36}

Life was beginning to improve. I had a job, though I was unsure if I would be able to keep it. I had a girlfriend, though she didn't live in the same city as me. I was moving to a new place soon, a huge loft in Midtown, and I had a roommate—Colin had gotten the internship, as expected, and I would be living with him—though he had not yet arrived. It was all coming together. But I remained unsure.

I passed my days clicking my mouse in fear, sitting in the open area of my office building, discussing across the monitors whether the document I was viewing looked responsive to the subpoena with one of the more experienced people on my project. If a privileged document, one which could be withheld due to attorney-client or work product privilege, walked out the door, I would be fired—this I knew. I hated the presence of attorneys, sometimes lurking in the background on a carbon copy line, altering the entire tone of the conversation. My clicking was as tentative as everything else. What if I was wrong? There was no room for mistakes. This had been made clear from the beginning, as if I didn't already know. But I would be leaving town again soon, so I only had to make it until then.

Tyler, another friend I'd grown up with, was getting married in a couple of weeks. He was a mainstay of my high school socialization and had participated in some of my college-related experiences as well. He had helped design and build a toilet chair that we made the summer after high school. It all began one day in July, when Tyler had discovered an abandoned toilet on the side of the road and picked it up. The next week, we spent a day dousing it with bleach, scrubbing it clean before toweling it off and spray painting it UVA blue and stenciling the Virginia "V" and its accompanying sabers in orange on the back of the bowl. Once the paint was dry the next day, we framed it on a sturdy square wooden base and attached wheels to it. It was meant to serve as a seat, while the tank could be used to store beer. It survived the duration of my UVA stay and remained in some underclassman's house in Charlottesville even after we left.

Tyler's Bronco not only delivered us the toilet that would become the college throne, it also provided the backdrop for my steeplechase pictures during mine and Shawn's return to Aiken from school. This memory had faded, but the framed picture still sat in my Atlanta apartment.

He was in so many of my stories of young adulthood—this wedding was to be a celebration of a friend's happiness as well as an opportunity to introduce Donna to my life from before. True to form, I could not or did not pay my own way; she bought the plane tickets using her frequent flyer miles.

"The only way I can buy them this way is to have you go through Chicago."

Atlanta to Chicago to Bentonville. This circuitous route would have to work, since I couldn't afford the direct route tickets. The manner in which I arrived was of little consequence to me anyway; I was far too excited about the opportunity to spend time with everyone, especially Tyler, whom I had not often seen. Our days as Aiken neighbors were over, and Tyler's oceanography studies put him out to sea for months at a time, eliminating the chance for contact with his land-locked friends, except during narrowly defined intervals. Even when such opportunities had come about in the past, I hadn't found the time to visit—work was too busy or the drive was too long for a weekend drop-in. Now that I had tasted isolation, I would not dwell there voluntarily, so I found my way to Bentonville.

This time it was different. I had a job, and I had a girlfriend. I was no longer the sideshow. I had it together, and I wouldn't have to talk solely about my wreck. There was something more. This would be fun and relaxing, and it was a reward of sorts for finally getting a job. Everyone would love Donna, and I felt certain that they would think her impressive.

The plane descended as I finished planning my weekend, and I glanced down at my day planner, where I had written Donna's flight information. Once I landed, she would be at my gate, and we would have to hurry to our next flight to finish our trip. The weather was clear, so we wouldn't run into a problem with flight cancellations. Everything was on schedule.

The plane continued its controlled descent when, without warning, my face began to ache, mildly at first, and then the pain increased exponentially. It was a sharp, searing pain that focused under my eyes. I tried to ignore it and relax. I had been through things like this before, though the site was new. I tried to accept that nothing was wrong, that it was just phantom nerve responses, my mind trying to create an incident where there was none. My subconscious was desperate to torment me with the past even when it was no longer relevant.

But the agony did not go away. I breathed through clenched teeth, and my eyes began to water as low groans escaped from my tightly sealed lips, my eyes squinting in a wince. I begged it to stop. Life wasn't about just me. This weekend was about something bigger than me. I was a spectator, tasked with showing up and shutting up. How hard could this be?

The squeak of the wheels signaled our arrival. My head was about to explode. This was an aneurysm. I was about to die. I wanted to run screaming from the plane, but I stayed seated until the captain turned off the "fasten seat belt" sign. I tried to calm myself down. I reminded myself that it wasn't an aneurysm, since I wouldn't have felt an aneurysm, and it felt like someone was stabbing me in the face with an ice pick. The doors opened, and I waited in line until it was my turn to exit.

Donna was waiting for me and waved as I approached, before she saw me up close, when her excitement turned to her standard empathy and concern.

"Hey, babe. How was your fli…what's the matter?"

"I don't know. I need to go to the bathroom. I'll be right back."

I ducked into a nearby restroom and ran cold water over my face to calm the panic. My face hurt like hell. It didn't fit any symptom that had ever described to me. I was going to die in an airport restroom in Chicago. I was still upset when I emerged from the bathroom.

"Something is really wrong. I feel like I am being stabbed in the face and my right ear is really hurting." My voice had become nasal as my watering eyes had brought the accompanying congestion.

"We need to get you to a hospital. Let's get to the front and have them call an ambulance. Can you carry your bag?"

We quickly made our way to the front of the airport, where I collapsed into a plastic seat in front of the doors for passenger pick-up, my face buried in my hands. The ambulance lights alerted everyone to the show, and they loaded me onto a stretcher. People stared. My face wouldn't stop hurting. This was simply a minor inconvenience, I told myself. Everything would be fine. I knew the pain would stop soon, and I just needed to calm down. I told myself that I was not going to die.

The ambulance arrived at the hospital, and I was hurriedly rushed out of the back on my stretcher and wheeled through the automated doors. With the successful handoff from the ambulance personnel to the hospital staff, I was wheeled down one of the halls to a bare, fluorescently lit room, where the flurry of activity slowed and I sat waiting my turn. The doctor entered a few minutes later, asking questions that I answered with the post-wreck tour. The pain had already begun to subside when the MRI showed I was fine.

"It appears to me that you are suffering from Barotitis. It usually occurs in divers or children and primarily causes ear pain. The pressure builds up behind the eardrum and causes pain until equilibrium is restored. In your case, since they had to rebuild your sinuses after your wreck, I suspect that this caused problems with the blood vessels in the region and did not allow them to effectively correct for the pressure imbalance. Before you fly, use Afrin to open up the passages, and you shouldn't have any other problems."

I wasn't going to die, but we were going to sleep in Chicago at a nearby hotel before leaving on the first flight to Fayetteville the next morning. We exited the hospital and grabbed the cab that had been called for us. With the next days' sunrise, my nasal cavity saturated with Afrin, the flight took to the air and landed without incident.

When I finally arrived in Bentonville, the story explaining my delay had already been widely circulated, and most of the people who approached me led with that topic. But conversations quickly moved to the wedding itself, then the stupidity of our collective youths, talk of our jobs, introductions to Donna, and discussions of future plans. The wedding took place, and the appropriate mood accompanied it. A group of kids dressed in the trappings of adulthood, laughing while holding our beers, was caught on film, wives and girlfriends in other shots, and the children at home. The pain, as always, was temporary, but the digital memory survived as a framed picture in my living room.

{chapter 37}

After I returned from Bentonville, I began again with a renewed sense of purpose. From that day forward, I lived at work, since my salvation had begun with my employment, and I planned to click my mouse on my way to success. I dreamt of my employer, so impressed with my coding, tapping me to resume partnership track employment at the main building. The concept was ludicrous, and they didn't even pretend that health insurance benefits were in my future.

Still, as time passed, I grew more and more comfortable. I made friends with many of my coworkers. My location made lunches with Chad and Susan easier, so we met with greater frequency. Colin moved in. Donna set an October date for when she would move down, and we adopted a dog together. My blood tests continued to come back negative.

I had finally outgrown my problems. Stability was sealing out chaos, and I grew accustomed to the order. I was still nervous about work, and the quality of my work product vacillated wildly as I struggled to maintain my concentration, with caffeine and boredom as the primary culprits for my insufficient attention span, but I noticed that some people began to ask for me on their projects. I drank to be social, not to escape. I hit safely in softball games. I attended trivia with Colin's friends from work, where my sports knowledge combined with others' knowledge of everything else to seal our victory. Though my confidence remained shaky, it continued to grow, and some days, my bluster even returned. I had learned enough. It was time to reap the rewards for my efforts.

I finally made the visit to New York in preparation for Donna's move. That Thursday, when the car that she ordered picked me up from the airport and took me to her building in the heart of Midtown Manhattan, I was amazed. The man at the front desk was friendly and confirmed my identity as someone allowed in. He passed me the key that Donna had left for me and gave me the apartment number so that I could drop my bags. I left for her work building three blocks away, looking up at the high-rise buildings all around me as I walked. Once I arrived, I stood in her lobby in front of security and waited for her to come down. The elevator opened, and she emerged. The weekend had begun.

I met her important friends, much as we had planned for before, and was amazed at their success. The first night, we had drinks with her friends at an upscale bar in one of the buildings close to her apartment. The next day I attended Donna's going away party at work and timidly stepped forward when I was recognized as the reason for her departure. Donna and I left for the country the following day to spend time with her best friend and her best friend's husband. I would try to engage him in a discussion of economic policy to show my intelligence before realizing that, just because I read The Economist, did not mean I could keep up with a Stanford M.B.A. on the subject. Everyone was friendly in their acceptance even as they saw how I did not measure up to what they were accustomed; since Donna was past the point of no return, in the spirit of friendship, they could only offer support. Once I arrived back in Atlanta, I sent Donna's famous boss flowers to thank her for allowing my girl to move down and readied for the importance that was about to descend on me.

In the evenings, I spent time with my brother as an adult, something I had never before had the opportunity to do. He was everything I wasn't: quiet, diligent and successful, the most impressive guy in most rooms he entered, but too modest to appreciate this fact. His girlfriend from school, Elizabeth, would visit almost once a month, and I watched them interact with great fascination. She was good for him, and he was growing into himself. She became his fiancé that Christmas break.

Mom met Donna's parents that Thanksgiving, and everyone got along in spite of their different backgrounds. Everything had come together. Aside from occasional rumblings of discontent at work from my bosses, intending to keep employees on our toes, there were no discordant sounds. My life was finally safe, and everything felt right.

I still noticed my weaknesses every day when, overwhelmed, I forgot an instruction or one of the tags or momentarily confused what agency our latest project was responding to in my hurry to start my work. But I had learned to pause and collect myself before the panic fully set in, and when my eyes returned to my screen, the information usually flooded back. No one mentioned anything to me about work issues. The days of fatal mistakes seemed behind me.

I was content. I eyed what others had with envy, but I reminded myself of the long hours and the inevitable failure that had accompanied my foray into a world outside of the one I now comfortably occupied. I didn't belong there anymore. I whined the normal whine of the low-level employee: no one respected me, my bosses sometimes acted like idiots, and everyone else received the credit while I did the work. I didn't like having people tell me what to do, especially since it lowered my standing in the eyes of others, but I knew the blame would seldom reach my pay grade, and I enjoyed my seemingly certain paycheck.

Once Donna arrived in Atlanta, she began to see my daily routine. I tried explaining to her that this might be as good as it would get, distorting and then adopting the mantra "know thyself," blind to the irony. But she didn't believe me, and I was finding that those around me had not abandoned my former dreams as rapidly as I had. Without prompting, they served as the proxy for my confidence while it remained hidden. Donna was the most forceful.

"I think you should at least look at some other jobs. Didn't Derek say he had contacts with some employment law firms? Did you talk to the man I emailed you about? Maybe he has heard of something out there that you would like to do."

Everyone else seemed to sense a discontent of which I was unaware. They heard my complaining and noticed changes in me. They saw my capabilities increasing gradually and witnessed those moments when it clicked, but they mistook these times as ordinary, and they missed the setbacks. They believed even while I did not. They thought I would soon outgrow my childish attachment to a world where failure was ridiculously unlikely, and I would soon seek out challenges, which I would then be armed to tackle.

I, on the other hand, knew this would not happen. The healing had probably stopped; I was most likely stuck with my new limitations. Aside from the ordinary problems of too much work and not enough pay, what was there to complain about? I ate lunch with Chad and Susan, went to Braves games with George, played intramural sports during the week, and I drank beers and watched football on my weekends. This was enough.

Even as my friends pushed me to look for something else and I refused, my comfortable world was becoming unsettled. Work came in by the truckload. Two million, one hundred thousand documents to review in five weeks. My employer instituted a bonus program to provide further incentive for all of the extra work, and I was at the office almost every waking hour, including weekends, knowing each extra hour provided additional pay that would help fund a lifestyle I hadn't fully forsaken, even as the money it required evaporated. I no longer had time for Donna and things were getting progressively worse between us already, but falling back on a prior failed strategy, I decided unilaterally that we could tackle the mounting list of issues once I finished with this project; work was too important to waste energy elsewhere.

I was too busy, completely overwhelmed, and choosing a negligibly larger paycheck over sleep, time with Donna, and intramural activities. When I had sent Jill's boyfriend Derek my resume at his request, I hadn't intended for the process to move so quickly, but in the middle of everything else, I headed to a scheduled morning interview, the first step toward a bigger dream others had for me.

"Derek speaks highly of you, and around here, that means a lot," the interviewing partner began.

I was tired and unsure, but this sounded as if I were a lock for the position.

"He had nothing but good things to say about your firm when I asked, so it seems the feeling is mutual," I replied.

The small talk continued before my unvanquished demons appeared.

"So, I see you started at Irwin Myers before you moved on to Cole Hyde."

"I guess that my employment history requires some explaining," I began, preparing to deliver The Excuse. "I know how it looks, with me starting at a big firm and now I am only doing document review work. I had a pretty bad car wreck just after I graduated, and I was in the hospital for about three months. It has taken me a while to recover, but I feel like my capabilities have finally returned, and I can do the work now."

He responded to my confession calmly.

"I don't see anything wrong with your current position. Derek mentioned to me that you were in a wreck. You still have a solid resume. I don't think that your explanation is necessary."

He hadn't terminated the interview, and he hadn't yelled at me for wasting his time. Honesty was certainly the way forward.

I moved to my next interview, where I discussed my volunteer work, the one thing I had to brag about, with a woman around my age. Instead of jumping at the opportunity to talk about these activities, I answered cautiously. I refused to sell myself, words of a past confrontation echoing in my head. I could remember only the bad in interviews. I knew, and they needed to know, that I was probably still broken.

The only story I was comfortable telling was the one about my wreck, so I brought it out unprompted during my other interviews, and the interviewer changed his or her questions and responses to accommodate me.

"Were you in a coma?"

"Does that cause problems when you're doing your job now?"

"It's amazing that you had to go through that."

I was making myself a human interest story on a job interview. I added soft light in the hopes that it would make the blemishes on the face of my resume disappear. But the relevant questions remained, and they were much harder to answer.

"Have you taken a deposition before?"

"Have you ever drafted a motion?"

"In your current position, do you have many opportunities to write?"

The answer was "no" to all of their questions. No, I didn't have any experience. No, I didn't know how to be a litigator. No, I didn't know why I was sitting in front of each of them, pretending I wanted the job they were offering.

My answer was simple, though I had no plans to give it. I had once sifted through boxes of worker's compensation claims while working for my current employer. I had seen how regimented this area of law was, and I thought I might be able to master this process with the aid of one of my organizational strategies. This was the best alternative I had.

I pondered all of this while my mouth provided a series of stock answers, highlighting what I had done in hopes they wouldn't see my uncertainty, which was not intended for their eyes. I finished the interviews back where I started. I thanked him for seeing me, and headed for the exits.

That afternoon, oblivious to how poorly the interviews had gone, I rode MARTA back to the office, hoping I hadn't gotten the job. I didn't know how to take a deposition, and I certainly didn't want to mess up something like that. My history was too littered with mistakes for me to risk another. For the last time, I had encountered a career obstacle with everything rigged in my favor, and failed to show the intestinal fortitude necessary to take what had been handed to me. Mediocrity was my fate, and the rejection letter the next week was a relief. I couldn't blame them. I would have gone a different direction, too.

{chapter 38}

"You will understand when you're my age."

I vaguely understood that day when she delivered her message. Donna was unhappy. That was why she was leaving. We had been going through the motions for long enough, an existence devoid of excitement, passion and energy. Our life together hadn't worked out. There were too many differences. This was not a mystery; it was a relationship ending. I hadn't been able to hold up my end of the bargain. She was tired of dealing with my daily exhaustion.

"You always have enough energy for the things you want to do," her email reminded me in the days that followed.

When I sat in my quasi-cube the next day and electronically coded the documents for the important client with an impossible deadline, with the huge cup of caffeine keeping me awake and the black cloud of adolescent despair hanging over my head, I thought I understood: she was tired of my limitations. The rest was diversionary chatter to distract me from this fact. It wasn't my fault. I was again being punished for my wreck, not by her, but by some cosmic force that dumped on me every day.

It wasn't until much later, long after the client thanked my superiors for our tireless efforts and after many more unsuccessful relationships, that I would finally arrive at a different conclusion. Maybe she was tired of sharing a bed with someone who did not dream her dream and kept hitting snooze. I would never become who she wanted me to be. Our trips to Savannah would never become vacations to France. My friends from kickball would never be named to corporate boards.

But there was a bigger problem. I wasn't becoming who I wanted to be, either. When would I finally face my problems and devise solutions? Our relationship, potentially doomed by our differences, had not deteriorated solely because I was tired. I had also actively poisoned it, with my dead-eyed moping and constant grumbling about my new reality, the one with no upside, an existence I had actively sought out when failure in any other venture still felt certain.

I had once known how to tackle the seemingly more difficult obstacles—the endless physical problems—simply because I'd had extensive experience with physical training from my younger days playing tennis, and I could see the results. If my balance was terrible, I stood on one foot while the elevator descended to the ground floor, I worked on my balance board at night, and I strengthened my core with thousands of crunches until it got better.

If I couldn't walk, I was never dissuaded by the rush of tile rising to meet me during repeatedly unsuccessful attempts. They had to tie me up to stop me from trying. Once I could walk, I had started to run, and once I was running, I had continued running farther and farther until my body failed me.

I loved telling my story, not just because it excused my lackluster life accomplishments, but also because, in a life where I was ashamed of almost everything, I was proud of what I had done. I had faced almost insurmountable obstacles, and overcome most of them. While I was busy polishing my story for maximum effect, I had forgotten the shin splints, the hallucinations, the face pain, the headaches, the frustrations, the night cage, and the loneliness of my hospital days. I had forgotten my silent promises and the need to fight to ensure that no failure was final. Disappointments at work were suddenly enough to stop my efforts completely. I had forgotten my blind belief that I would eventually be successful. I was sitting stationary, waiting for handouts. I had forgotten the lessons I had sworn I would never forget.

Maybe that's what everyone saw as they pushed me to reach for more. Donna had been willing to participate in my reclamation project, but she expected forward movement, and likely an arrival at a destination that I could never reach. She had jet-setting friends and desired the lifestyle they participated in; she would not bind herself to a financially unsuccessful guy who whined but accepted his fate.

I thought that those extra hours at work had been to buy me time, to show that I could still afford the successful life—a last request for an extension on my assignment. Instead, she had seen it for what it was: as surrender, an acceptance of a life I viewed as mediocre. I had once been so promising. I was supposed to emerge more rapidly than this. I was supposed to keep trying. I was supposed to stop failing.

She had run out of patience with wasting her life anchored to someone who stubbornly refused to keep believing and who had resigned himself to a fate he did not want; so she took the dog and left. We remained in contact and, following a familiar pattern, the dog was the centerpiece of our electronic correspondence, but she never discussed the precise reasons why it ended, so I'll never know. I know being with me required her to sacrifice things to which she had previously grown accustomed, like world travel, and she finally tired of making these sacrifices. But my unwillingness to keep going is why I would have left me.

Only now do I understand why I hated me.

{chapter 39}

The revelations of tomorrow are never useful today. I wasn't ready to jump into action. It hadn't even been four years, and I had too much left to observe, so I passively continued on.

Colin was getting married, and he made me his best man. I was closer with him than I had been in years, due to our daily contact the year that he worked in Atlanta. Before this, we had not been as close as we were growing up. Once I left for college, we had never lived near each other again and, since neither of us was comfortable talking on the phone for long periods of time, our contact had been extraordinarily limited before our year living together.

Though our interaction had changed in nature as it increased in frequency, one part of our dynamic had not changed during our year as roommates: I very much viewed him with a tempered form of reverence, despite the fact he was my junior. I had always seen him as my intellectual superior, but with Elizabeth's guidance, his social skills were beginning to surpass mine, as well.

I knew I needed to make the bachelor party perfect, because that's what he deserved, and I spent the weeks before his wedding researching our options. I didn't know all of his friends on the guest list well, though I'd met most of them at least once or twice, and I polled the group to see what might interest everyone. First, we considered renting a boat for deep sea fishing, but it was prohibitively expensive. Golf was out, since he infrequently played the sport. Slowly, the options melted away, and my epic endeavor had been reduced to what I could manage, and even then I feared that I wouldn't pull it off successfully, since I was planning the bachelor party in a city where I did not reside.

The envisioned elaborate production was reduced, at his request, to a night out in Virginia Beach and the accompanying bachelor party festivities, which most of his invitees would be able to make. I hoped it would be enough, that it was in fact what he wanted, not simply an arbitrary "three rating" for his bachelor party planning scorecard. The plan in place, I focused on coordinating rides for the arriving guys in my Excel spreadsheet.

That Wednesday, my flight arrived, and with my rental car full of people I had met only a couple of times, I drove to our evening's destination, listening to them banter about work and college and observing the dynamic of a group my brother had participated in during the years after childhood.

Once we arrived and parked the car, everyone gathered at the hotel. It had been a success. Everyone was there. The rest of the plan was on autopilot and no longer required my strict observation. Relieved, I picked up a beer, and made it an hour into the night before I blacked out.

The next day, no worse for wear, I finished the drive to Elizabeth's parents' house and everyone in the car laughed about the previous evening, much of which I had not been privy to. When we got to Colin's soon-to-be in-laws' house, we played volleyball in their backyard with even more people I did not know. The rehearsal dinner was at a nearby seafood restaurant and was the precursor to the union of two families. Colin's friends talked while the families mingled. Elizabeth's father and I discussed a recent Supreme Court decision regarding the permissibility of a strip search of a student in a high school, not typical conversation at such an event, but he was a vice principal at a school and I masqueraded as a lawyer, so he talked about what he knew, and I pretended that I knew more than I did.

{the detours}

The next day, I watched Colin get married. Mom smiled through her tears, and I stood at the front while they exchanged their vows, thinking about how much time had passed. My little brother was six-foot-three, would finish medical school the next year, and was about to walk out a married man. Smartly attired, I had seen it all up close, and I was watching the skinny kid who had once read books during his tennis match change-overs leave for good.

Once we arrived at the reception, I nervously sipped on the Crown Royal my cousin Jazz's husband had snuck in and prepared to congratulate them for doing what I had not: for finding happiness and becoming adults together.

I took a deep breath as I rose, pinging my fork against my glass of champagne. My nerves, as always, were shot. The frozen fear born of my awkward goodbye to Eric, of Amy walking out the door before I could describe my appreciation for her sacrifices, of every one of my missed opportunities to explain to others the momentousness of an occasion, flashed ever so briefly in my head before the practiced words crowded out the worst of the unease.

I tried to slow my speech and take my time. This was important. I needed to say goodbye to my brother as the quiet kid brother from childhood who I once suplexed off the living room couch, and explain to them that I understood, at least vaguely, who he had become, before wishing both him and Elizabeth well in their next step of adulthood. With all eyes on me, I heard my voice, tinged with nervous pride.

"I have always admired the way my brother effortlessly accomplishes so much. This year, I have had the opportunity to live with him and discovered that he is a good softball player; can knock back beers when the situation calls for it; is, in fact, much bigger than I am (as intuitive as that is for most, I'm still coming to grips with it); and knows more about medicine, due to the countless medical journals that he reads, than anyone who hasn't been practicing for a decade.

"I met Elizabeth after Laura Carlson's wedding. Unbeknownst to me, my date asked her what she did. When Elizabeth answered, 'I'm a nurse,' this woman responded, 'How cliché,' since she knew Colin was studying to be a doctor. About six months later, when Elizabeth told me this story, two things I already knew were confirmed: Elizabeth was a keeper and my date to the wedding was not."

The crowd laughed, and Colin and Elizabeth smiled. They all understood that I knew the people who were sitting in front of us, that I was part of their family and would be forever. I felt the rush of relief. Colin and Elizabeth were still happy. I hadn't ruined their moment. I knew it was time to finish my goodbye, to return to the anonymity where I felt most comfortable.

"I have appreciated the opportunity to get to know Elizabeth better over this past year when she and their dog Lundy would visit Atlanta. I knew her to be smart and hard-working, as working while going to school part-time has shown. She has demonstrated remarkable maturity around me while still remaining fun to be around. Most importantly to me, she makes my brother happy. Join me as I raise my glass to wish Elizabeth and Colin a happy and prosperous life together. I know that with both of your abilities, it is inevitable."

With that, my duties were finished, and my tension vanished. The champagne disappeared and my beer was empty by the end of the maid of honor's speech, so I walked to the bar to pick up my next serving. People came up to me to tell me how much they enjoyed the toast, and by the time I returned to the table to resume talking with my cousins, I was content, knowing I had successfully played my part. I looked around and saw familiar faces from my time in Aiken, talking and laughing. I soaked in my brother's happiness. This was good enough.

{chapter 40}

"Get over yourself… maybe you would be happier then."

Even over email, Brooke's command snapped with contempt. Four months after my successful efforts for Colin's wedding, I heard the tired refrain of my life once again: it was another failed relationship. This had all begun with a chance encounter in Charlottesville at a leadership conference.

When I had left for Charlottesville five months prior, life was not bleak in any sense of the word. It was mildly uncomfortable but distinctly monotonous. My week days remained formulaic. Wake, code, sleep. When the yelling at work started, it was always in a group setting so that I would wonder if it was my work at fault and push myself harder, if only for a few brief days, until I once again tired of the drudgery. Did they see mistakes that I was missing? I couldn't tell, and one day I was coding too slowly, the next too carelessly, but never just right.

I couldn't begin to calm down until I stopped hearing their amorphous criticism, and even when that stopped, I took their silence as rejection of my work. My fear was knowing precisely what I could never have happen again—another quiet pink slip graciously slipped to me wrapped in an apology—and feeling it around every corner. All of my senses sought it out, some distorting the ordinary just to find it.

I knew I wasn't learning a skill, but the goal was simply to keep receiving a paycheck, nothing more. I didn't have time or energy for anything else during the week, except occasional softball games, since the coffee began to fade by late afternoon and the coding frequently continued even after its departure. I emailed with my work friends throughout the day to break up the monotony and spent large quantities of time exchanging witticisms with a coworker, Carrie, with whom I had struck up a random political conversation at work one day. The firm still gave me most of my weekends. Life hadn't been bad.

The weekends had been a completely different story, as my newest work friend, Dustin Irwin, personified fun with a cocktail in hand. I sat around his place with the games on TV and a beer in hand, or followed him around the late night bars, watching him approach total strangers and strike up a conversation. He was at ease in social situations, brimming with confidence, and most weekends he was in his element a couple of drinks down. When he invited me, I followed him. The parts of his life in which I participated were fun, and, thus, by association, so was mine.

My trip to Charlottesville that random weekend was simply to be another weekend distraction from the daily grind, much like my bar hopping with Dustin, except using locations from college. This Charlottesville experience had been a disorienting trip, first involving a chance encounter with a former pledge class member, and with this meeting, feeling the accompanying residual social awkwardness from college.

Then, as I was preparing for the final celebratory dinner our last night in town, I found myself holding one of the lenses to my glasses in my left hand and my glasses' frame in my right. I would go through the evening legally blind, but a second chance encounter, this one with a female officer by the name of Brooke, of the UVA Club of Chicago, provided additional opportunities for time away from my reality. Our Charlottesville encounter, limited both in duration and in sensory data, supplied enough intrigue that I did not hesitate to chase her through my electronic lifelines.

The reality I continued to flee had evolved as time progressed. My stock portfolio, the future down payment for when I found Mrs. Right and she wanted the symbols of material success, had taken a beating as the market began its steep descent, confirmed by an ever-gloomier Bloomberg website automatically updating in the background. The ship was sinking. My friend from my second job, George, who only a few months before had taken a chance and left for a small law firm specializing in sophisticated real estate exchanges intended to preserve wealth, wondered aloud how much longer he would have a job. Chad sat in his office with little to do as the credit markets began to freeze.

I ignored it all. Brooke had come to Atlanta and sung karaoke with my friends. I had visited Charlottesville, met her parents, and watched UVA lose horribly to USC with her and Shawn Carlson and his girlfriend. Brooke invited me to Chicago, where I had seen The Second City and watched the Cubs clinch the pennant, and I had toasted the Cubs' success in the bars of Wrigleyville with intoxicated strangers. My weekend life with her had been perfect.

The problem had been the work weeks in between. Though my job wasn't horrible, I still didn't enjoy it, nor was there a future at the firm, and my age-old fear that I was soon to be fired cropped up with far too much regularity. Some days I could convince myself it was all in my head, but mere minutes after the next meeting that outlined our group errors, I was back in a funk for the subsequent week. I overwhelmed Brooke with my worries and my insecurities in my daily emails, and she continued on with her seemingly carefree life in Chicago, occasionally worrying in print that my lack of spontaneity and morose outlook on life would drag her down and destroy whatever we had. Her interest began to wane as my panic took control and, after a confusing email exchange, Chicago was no longer the electronic destination for my passive hopes for a better tomorrow. I was left to get over myself in Atlanta.

{chapter 41}

No longer effectively distracted, I turned to look at what I had built. There wasn't much to observe. I was another year older but still had few discernible job skills, and there were no longer resumes circulating, since I had no plans to change anything. I lived in unsettled mediocrity. I felt stronger than before, but that could have been those extra morning cups of coffee I'd been consuming. My balance was better, my left hand almost worked as it should, and I hadn't had one of those horrible headaches in months.

The final reminders of yesterday's unpleasantness began to make their curtain calls. A white spot randomly appeared along my gum line, and after prodding it for a few weeks, I visited the dentist to have it looked at. It was a small part of my jaw that had splintered off during the wreck. One day it had unexpectedly moved away from its original resting place, masked deep within my gums next to the jaw's point of impact with the car dashboard. It had finally surfaced along my gum line to form the white spot I then noticed, and so I visited my dentist to see what could be done about it. When it was jerked free by a dental assistant and shown to me, I saw a white bone chip resembling a piece of a dove from a broken sand dollar. The other scars from my wreck had already faded into the background to such a degree that they were barely visible even if I tried to point them out, and, free of the debris, my gums healed over, leaving no additional indications of past trauma. There was nothing left to commemorate my ignominious fall from grace.

By now, almost everything around me had changed. I had held Chad's daughter at the hospital the day after she was born and watched her blink tiny eyelids adorned with fractional eyelashes before returning to sleep. Colin and Elizabeth were headed to New Haven, where he was to complete his residency at Yale, and I spread the word to all who would listen, my pride in my brother obvious. I had been in George and Renee's wedding in Charleston and they had been in their new house for over a year when he was laid off. The job market was horrible, so he went out on his own, opening his own practice with Renee's help. Everyone was finding their way.

With no solution to my daily consternation readily apparent, I instead found myself on a plane to New Orleans, where I would be staying with Shawn and Brooke Carlson, who were married in Hawaii a few weeks after my visit to Charlottesville, and meeting up with law school friends for Mardi Gras. My itinerary was full of events, and I felt the pulse of the city as the plane touched down. I sought to divide my time between Shawn and my law school friends. Despite the hurricane the city had weathered two years before, the Midtown area still looked as I remembered it, and the subtle differences around me were not enough to dissuade me from immediately falling into character. I had tried to grow up. I had tried to plan out my life, and my planned life rejected me. I was once again going to be fun. It was time to reclaim my youth.

That weekend the beer flowed freely, and the adrenaline rush never stopped. It felt like Vegas—I was with people I had rarely seen since graduation, some, like Joel, close friends I only sporadically saw in person due to distance, and some of them people I considered friends from school but had otherwise not kept up with. As the blur began, I basked in the warm numbness of the moment. I wandered the streets during the day, and G Love played me to bed at night. I dressed myself in maturity as we all headed to Commander's Palace for brunch, and my jacket hid the stains as I poured yet another twenty-five cent martini down the front of my blue shirt.

{pulling off the road}

There, in front of me, she of law school fame, one of the desired, sat and laughed at my stories, and I continued to talk, accelerating the words as if I had answers or had discovered cleverness at the bottom of the last glass while I refreshed my shirt with the next. The laughter echoed in my head even after we had left the closed confines of the restaurant. It was the timbre of my youthful dreams. The spirit of the moment, carefree and borderline reckless, combined with cocktails to fuel the remainder of the day and changed my evening's destination.

Waking in a hotel room that wasn't mine next to the golden-haired object of my desire, I was amazed at my good fortune and immediately began to consider ways I could freeze that moment, to preserve it so that I could revisit it—and the adrenaline and endorphins it supplied—well into the future. As I walked to meet Shawn, I felt accomplished, my acceptance by the world to which I still wished to return no longer in doubt. I prepped for the day of parades with countless cocktails at our pre-parade rendezvous, and as the day hurried toward night, I got lost in the bars chasing my fantasy.

The darkness found me incoherent and confused, wandering half-empty Midtown streets barefoot with a useless sandal in hand and my toe blackened and broken from my fall down the steep Balcony Bar stairs just minutes before. My evening's goals, once ambitious and lustful, were replaced by the desperate desire to locate Shawn's house and call it a night. I didn't understand how a once-promising day had fallen apart so fast. After I walked a mile in the wrong direction and turned around to complete the return trip with Shawn's telephonic guidance, I finally achieved my more manageable aim.

The next morning, Shawn and I were eating breakfast at a nearby diner before I left for the airport.

"I know you were seeing your law school friends and getting away from Atlanta, but I think you may want to take it easy.

You were ridiculously drunk this weekend. Maybe you shouldn't drink so much," he suggested.

I flinched at the criticism while I moved another forkful of my omelet to my mouth before beginning my guarded response. "Yeah, I guess I got out of control. I needed to get away so badly that I turned off my self-control when I left. I don't usually drink that much."

And with that, the Defense rested. Two sentences later, we were discussing the city and his plans, his painfully honest observation in the past, not to be dredged up again.

But she responded to my text that morning. There was no reason to dwell on the methodology when the results were so readily apparent. The texts were precursors to emails, the emails to conversations, and the conversations became visits. I would successfully escape reality again. I was the Harry Houdini of life.

This time, though, the escape wasn't as clean. My toe was broken, though this was the least of my concerns. The fantasy world to which I had escaped was growing less and less tolerant of my behavior. I had wasted an opportunity to spend quality time with Shawn, with Amy, and with Joel, opportunities I rarely had, all because I wouldn't grow up. Everyone was tiring of dealing with a stunted adolescent. They saw me as whole once again, and they felt no need for continued leniency. The excuses were getting old.

"At the end of the day, the bigger concern for me (and while this is dangerous pot-kettle territory for me, I feel that it should be stated) was the fact that you seemed hell-bent on drinking yourself into oblivion at every turn without any interest in any social interaction," Joel's email read. "While we all tend to get there eventually, it is better not to do it by 10am, or to lap the field twice. I know you have some social anxiety, but you can't always compensate for that by getting black-out wasted. I don't know what the solution is for you, but it needs to be addressed."

Joel's email and its honest observations, couched in the vocabulary of friendship, were an indictment of my coping scheme and spoke of solutions, but I felt that it was too soon. The job market remained a desolate wasteland, devoid of opportunity, so I didn't see how I could change my life. I felt that I needed to survive until tomorrow, when I would finally have a chance to make the necessary changes. I was still inside my five-year window on healing, so buying time meant I was getting stronger. And she was interested in me despite my issues. There still had to be some redeemable qualities present.

I noted everyone's input and promised myself that I would return to it at a future time when I could do something about it. Until then, I would keep my head down and soldier on. I continued to spend copious amounts of time at work, and my apparent usefulness gave me meaning, with evening breaks for sporting events or beers with Carrie and weekend breaks for travel or bars when I didn't have to work.

I emailed her of New Orleans fame, and she became Julie while I remained paranoid—of being fired, of her becoming disinterested, of never finding my way. I tried to hide it most days, but the incessant barrage of messages that I dispatched made it clear that I could not find fulfillment independent of someone else.

Viewing people as answers may not have been healthy for either party involved, but it was sufficient for me, since I had long ago given up the hope that I would ever arrive on my own, and I still needed to feel as if I remained productive with my daily activities. Therefore, my emails became a search for a better future, more fun than job hunting yet, in my mind, just as necessary. I couldn't do this alone; I needed someone else to be there with me.

I travelled to Washington, D.C., and met her friends and spied on her life. She was fun, and so were her friends. I knew they had their own concerns, their own gnawing doubts, but they could interact and not reveal them with every syllable like I did. They knew how to enjoy life, and I hoped it would become contagious. Then, on the last day I was there, as we walked around the Georgetown area of D.C. and enjoyed the still mild temperatures, I started to hear my reality in her life.

"You know, couples that have two salaries, if one of them gets fired, they can still live off the other person's."

There it was. Julie buried it, unthinkingly, in a throw-away sentence in a meandering conversation. We were all searching for stability and for security, and it would never be enough. None of us ever had enough money in the bank or would be completely insulated from the fears of career termination. Julie was bright and, from the stories of her daily interactions, I assumed well-respected at work. She was a federal government employee, protected from arbitrary termination by mountains of regulations, offered a government pension plan and federal health insurance, and all of these things had kept her fears quiet initially.

I was an at-will employee who was only tolerated at the office, without benefits, and always one illness away from medical bills that would drain everything I had in savings. Yet we both sought the same security and, though I couldn't tell what price she was willing to pay for it, it had definitely influenced her career choice and, from what I heard that day, it would inform her choice regarding the individual she would date and perhaps marry. We were both chasing absolute safety and, though she was much closer to catching it, it still looked unlikely that she would ever be able to do so.

I incorporated the new input as rapidly as possible, but only so far as my interactions with her were concerned. When she made the reciprocal journey to meet me in Atlanta, I presented Chad, Valerie, and their daughter. I had proof I was a stable choice. My friends were married but still fun. I always hinted that the job security would come later when the economy improved, for now I was still getting stronger. The audition was going well.

But situations came up in the interim, and I assumed the worst. She got sick with a respiratory condition and stopped communicating with me as frequently, and her silence chastised me for my weaknesses, for my inability to converse properly with her friends, for my unimpressive career, for my daily awkwardness, and for everything that I was not. I heard her voice whispering to me what I had been repeating in my head for years. Her daily concerns in D.C. were not appropriate explanations for her moments of inattentiveness. I was struggling to overcome things that no one understood, facing virtually unimaginable hurdles, yet she didn't spend her waking time concerned with my well-being? She clearly wasn't interested in me. My neuroses won. By the time my birthday arrived, we were friends, the kind who never speak.

{chapter 42}

I continued to seek out distractions but no longer found anyone willing to play the game with me. They had their own problems and their own realities to face. Chad had been laid off early in the year, since my one-time employers had analyzed their economic models and determined that the market for his services would not return soon enough to justify his continued paycheck. He and Valerie would soon move to Louisiana, somewhere he could secure a job. Thanks to the economy, Susan had been let go, as well, and was searching for work. George was hard at work establishing his practice. I was the only one running.

There were no more trips to postpone tomorrow. My meaning was finally tied to Atlanta, even while many of my friends scattered to other cities or began to spend their free time fighting to preserve their jobs. Work slowed, as our clients became more cost-conscious and postponed their day of reckoning and the legal bills it would entail. I was left to question my utility, as the institutional affirmation was replaced with more virulent reminders of how our inactivity was a product of our inadequacies. As always, I internalized it all. The mood grew somber around the office and emails with friends reflected a renewed terror of termination.

The institution that had thrice rejected me as a candidate for promotion did not appear to be softening its stance, and many of the individuals for whom I had once worked looked elsewhere for help on their projects. It appeared there was a long and arduous road in front of me, and so, after sporadic assignments and plummeting billable hours, I finally began to venture out of my comfort zone, sometimes proactively and sometimes at the direction of others.

I worked diligently gathering evidence and speaking to all of the interested parties trying to resolve the intractable issues of the custody dispute for which I served as a guardian ad litem. In furtherance of my duties, I made occasional visits to get to know the children and understand their habits and present living situation, observing her artistic bent in her most recent school endeavor, which hung proudly on the fridge, or watching him race his Hot Wheels cars around his elevated track.

The final visits took place, and I spent our last afternoon sitting at the Olive Garden, discussing school and life with two hyper individuals who were half my height while they picked at their chicken fingers. Despite the enormity of the decision I would soon have to make, I did not feel overwhelmed. Instead, I calmly sat in the booth in front of them, shepherding them back from the edge of the bench while listening to them tell their directionless stories that captured their typical days. The renewing power of working with forever optimistic kids, who were somewhat aware yet undaunted by the hardness of life, made me forget my dull day and the unending aches of existence. It was only supposed to be a project that I volunteered for during work's slowest months to fill time while giving a little back. But I had become emotionally entangled, and had been desperately trying to find a resolution to their dilemma since the end of January.

I asked to help on a volunteer project tasked with obtaining disability benefits for wounded veterans, and we seemed to be making a difference. I was assigned to another pro bono project where I highlighted deposition testimony to prepare for the firm's case defending a death row inmate.

During this manufactured industriousness, I was robbed of the kind words of my employer, since the beneficiaries of my efforts did not pay our bills and my efforts did not register on the spreadsheet that mattered to my superiors. I felt the malaise began to lift, and it was replaced with righteous indignation. How much money had Chad made our former employer before they tossed him away? How sincere was the sales pitch that lured George away from his more established position? Did Susan's twenty-five years of service not mean anything? What would stop my employer from treating me the same way? How many of my friends would have to be discarded before I finally understood?

Carrie and I formed a closer connection at work through continued email banter during the day, and our regular conversations continued to amuse me and helped suppress my growing rage at the perceived callousness of my employer. We discussed the day's happenings outside of work over beers or at hockey or some other sporting event, like we had done for the last two years, but I finally began to wonder aloud what I had yet to internalize: this was a business, so why wouldn't my bosses simply make business decisions?

Perhaps the reason I had been passed over for promotion was that my attitude was horrible, and my work product was average. Some of my bosses still likely questioned my aptitudes, but far more noticeable was my immaturity. I possessed the coping skills of an adolescent, and I wore my unhappiness defiantly, as if it were someone else's job to fix this problem, and their unwillingness to address the concern in a timely manner meant I had been wronged.

And so I stood, faced with a reality I heartily despised, again dressed as a martyr on the way to my execution. It wasn't fair. I was supposed to be better than this; I was supposed to be whole by now. I had done my time. I had put in my five-plus years. Where was my reward? Why hadn't it gotten better?

"I think you are as strong now as you were before the wreck."

Hadn't that moved from a minority opinion held by a delusional mother to a consensus view shared by friends and acquaintances alike? They couldn't all be wrong, could they?

Yet I remained rooted to the spot. Dustin, my social proxy, left to pursue his career ambitions in another town. This did not sway me; instead, I spent more time hanging out with Jill's boyfriend Derek, joining him for beers after work while debating NBA or NFL team loyalty. I remembered the past selectively, and I would not forget the symptoms of my still present condition. I could not return to unemployable, pathetic, broken kid without prospects, begging for a sideways glance, hopeful that some company would show me pity. My present lot in life was all I would get. Contentedness was the secret to survival, and my inability to master it was a contributing reason why I had been passed over for promotion. If I could learn this simple concept, everything would be okay.

Once again, I had spent the holidays grumbling about everything, but I had returned to work determined to demonstrate leadership and industriousness, to finally meet my work superiors' expectations. As the business world once again began showing signs of life, the projects began to trickle back in, and I hoped the employer affirmation I needed would return with it. But I was assigned to a non-billable project that required a far greater mastery of legal research, technological know-how, and group coordination than anything with which I had previously been tasked. I poured myself into it, hoping this could differentiate me from others—that I could finally earn the respect for which I so desperately yearned.

Instead, it showcased my inefficiency, my efforts taking far longer than was expected. I tried to juggle my billable assignments with the more challenging unbillable task to which I'd also been assigned, all while the concluding hearings for my child custody case were taking place—an action that was finally drawing to a close with the final drops of venom spilled in transparent attempts to influence my recommendation to the Court.

I felt as overwhelmed as I had almost three years before, when I had begun. The self-doubt began to creep in again; my gasconade disappeared as the timidity returned. I still couldn't handle this job, really. How could I honestly still aspire to do something more? I was 30 years old. It was time to put away my daydreams. I had work to do. I was hundreds of hours off my billable pace. As the requests for my weekends resumed, I remembered what I had tethered myself to and learned the price of my security.

the
trip
resumes

{chapter 43}

It itched, and it wouldn't leave me alone. Aspiring to be more was noble, wasn't it? I was supposed to be content with my professional life, and I wasn't. But monotony, the safety of the daily repetition—that's where I could successfully live. I could learn to ignore the sting of others' implicit superiority. My mind would eventually drop the visions of the unattainable dream, just like it did everything else. I didn't really understand what this dream looked like, anyway. This job was where I belonged. There was nothing wrong with it. I was lucky. Hadn't I seen what happened to my friends who had ventured out? Had I already forgotten the days when I would have given anything to calm the confusion? This was the best I could do. I was happy outside of work. I needed to learn to be content.

I tried to get Carrie to sign off on this one evening just down the street over our usual Miller Lights. She had been a friend more so than a coworker from the moment we began working just down the hall from one another, and we had slowly transitioned to more. She had heard my stories, and she had watched my struggles. I shared with her, not to impress her, but to sort out events verbally before I could do so silently. We had played over email for years. She knew me far better today than anyone else in my life, and I trusted her.

For that reason, I was now looking to her for that external affirmation I'd always sought, confirmation that my vision was clear and that my solution was the right one. If she would simply say yes, I could dismiss the nagging feeling and bury it in a place where I wouldn't have to see it again for at least a few decades, when I could address it with the regret of a proud man reminiscing about youthful follies. I would be free of delusional dreams, and I could grumble the vision-hungry rumble of the scared—of those with too much to lose to venture out. I could invert the process and acquire the necessary elements to affirm my conclusions after the fact.

They were natural steps, anyway. I wanted a wife. I wanted a mortgage. I didn't want to have to think about why I was doing anything; I just wanted to do it. I was so tired of fighting an unwinnable fight against my limitations, whether they were physical, personal or professional. I only needed her permission, and I could be temporarily free of my final major problem: a continued desire to dream big while acting small. I took a swig from the bottle and told Carrie, for the last time, that I could not justify the risk of leaving, a risk I had discussed with her ad nauseam, and I waited for her agreement. If she would sign off on it, I would be done.

She shrugged instead, and with that shrug, everything changed. The pattern would not continue with her. She would not help me postpone the day of reckoning, and she would not pretend that she might be willing to make my important life choices for me. The decisions were mine to make because it was my life, and it was time to take ownership of them. If I asked her opinion, I would not receive the blind affirmation I was searching for. She would vocalize her opinion when it was requested and continue to challenge me, even if I simply wanted the easy answer. She was willing to support me when I needed her, but I had to learn to stand on my own and face the challenges as they arose.

"Tomorrow, would you regret not being a document review attorney anymore?" she asked. "Would you really miss being like everyone else, being their cog?"

Yes, my mind answered quickly. Even before making the decision, I could feel the regret. I had to work so hard to get there. I was useful there. I fit there. I just wanted to be like everyone else. I didn't want to be noticeably damaged anymore, and I could hide there. I wanted to blend in. I wanted safety.

But I already chafed against the weekly threats of firing, especially as they grew louder and less subtle. Safety, always illusory, was no longer even being proffered. Even if it had been, I wouldn't have wanted it at the exclusion of everything else tomorrow; at that moment, I was already beginning to question whether I wanted this safe life anymore. I could already feel the pull of something bigger. There was no mortgage that had to be paid. There was no wife demanding a stable future. There were no kids to feed, no expensive school tuitions to pay. I was a prisoner only to my own fear, an illogical apprehension of the unknown fueled by my previously unsuccessful attempts.

I had forgotten too much already. I didn't want memories of a big dream to disappear too, not yet. I wanted to spend my life watching this dream grow. Someday, reality might kill it, maybe even in its infancy, but I didn't want to watch it die at my hands.

I went home and slept on it every night for a week. Every day I returned lacking the conviction I possessed the night before—daylight again supplied the paralyzing terror. That final day, I came in to the office and began my routine anew. But this time, clicking my mouse was no longer sufficient. I needed words.

The email that appeared on my screen would serve as my two-week notice. I was seconds away from quitting a job. Countless other people had done this very thing. It wasn't unique. For me, though, I was about to embrace uncertainty for the first time, and it was as terrifying as I imagined.

I considered all of my options one last time and then clicked "Send." As the email vanished from my screen, for one second, before the resulting worries and problems had a chance to make their inaugural visit, I was completely in control of my own destiny. The serenity that had always flitted just out of reach, emerged from a haze of nerves, and I finally felt its relief.

{chapter 44}

I arrive in the present, a date much later on the calendar than I had intended—time stealthily crept along while I was looking back. The final period of this book will be pressed into service over seven years from the day of my wreck. I am thirty-two. I invested the final months of age 30 and all of age 31 assembling the history you now hold. Those months of scavenging for scraps of information, asking questions to which I should have known the answers, reliving the cringe-inducing dark days through hospital documents, police reports, emails, and interviews with others, and frenetically typing words I refused to save, all resulted in a new identity.

Is this enough to sustain me? I have had to pay yesterday's bills with tomorrow's funds, and if I remain tentative about what I've learned, I know that redemption will remain as elusive as ever. The money is gone, and I've used up the patience of those around me. Seven years have passed, and I will never get them back. For seven years, other people learned a number of things: how to do their jobs, how to live their lives, how to love their mates, how to dream. I have spent much of those seven years collecting experiences that I'm not sure I even remember, and occasionally arriving at important conclusions, only to misapply them. It took me all seven years to realize that sometimes I needed to remember where I had been; but sometimes, it was best to forget.

The mundane did not survive the synopsis, but even in the midst of my ongoing identity crisis, life was frequently enjoyable, and even the lows could be educational. But I have now finally arrived in the promised land of today and have the opportunity to alter tense, to type without knowing how the action will resolve or what hardships the next page will bring.

Every day the memories get fuzzier, and the harder I try to hold on, the faster they leave me, like individual grains of sand falling through my clenched fist. It's time to just let go. I have lost too much to discern exactly what once was, and today I lost more, just as I will tomorrow, too. But there are many things that I have learned by dwelling on my past, and in my head, for all these months and for far too many years before I made it a full-time endeavor. I have great friends and an amazing family. I don't deserve them, and I never will. I have done many things for which I am ashamed, and I have run from far too many challenges and stood crying in the face of others. I did not live up to my own expectations since, with the selfless support I have received, I know I could have accomplished more. But fleeing my mistakes does not absolve me of any responsibility, and blaming one unintended event for all of my pain does not soothe the hurt.

I'm sick of living with guilt for the talents I wasted, for the opportunities I squandered, and for my inadequacies as a friend, as a brother, as a son and as a significant other. I'm tired of being disappointed about things I cannot change and passive about things I can. I'm embarrassed that I'm not in better shape, that I'm not more mature and that I'm not more well-read, when I have spent the last seven years focusing on me, frequently to the exclusion of every other person in my life and my relationships with them.

Am I today manufacturing epiphanies that have not been realized? Having struggled so mightily to create these pages of memories and pseudo-memories mimicking a normal person's past, am I unwilling to accept the hollowness of the accomplishment? Am I now simply trying, in these final paragraphs, to justify an existence predicated on unfulfilled promise and once dominated by a pain so real that it can no longer be precisely identified? Was this simply one last backward-looking obsession before I could continue trudging ahead, blaming everything else for the bad while taking the lion's share of credit for the meager accomplishments?

I don't think so. There will always be remnants of these fears in the background—the disgust I once harbored for my present identity cannot, in an instant, be discarded when it was once so dominant an emotion, and it will probably always contribute in some small way to my motivations. But the need to explain the bad times away, to relegate my past to the past where it does in fact belong, but where I cannot even choose to visit it to find strength or revisit a piece of my identity, is finished.

I am sorry if this entire exercise seems self-indulgent. I'm sorry I have spent my life fixating on two unfortunate events in an existence defined by prosperity and opportunity. I'm sorry for the things that I did in my past that hurt people, regardless of whether I remember the events in question. I'm sorry if a story created from my recollections, journal entries, hundreds of emails and the memories of others, wounds anyone who remembers this time differently. I have done what I am willing to do to protect everyone. I'm sorry, but that is my last apology until the inevitable day when my future conduct renders another one appropriate. Until then, there will be no more.

My story, first told so many years ago—when I was ignorant of too many facts and single-minded in my need to apologize for who I wasn't—was one focused exclusively on two days of an occurrence, the impact of which will span all my remaining years, and has now finally become what I always needed it to be: a search for a new identity, different than the one I previously possessed yet informed by memories of the guy I once was.

It is time to recognize the new reality. This is my life. I'm not borrowing it from a friend. It is mine, and I am proud of it. I will no longer apologize for what it looks like to others. I could have made it different, perhaps better, perhaps worse. The detours were my path, despite the fact it was not the journey I initially intended. No matter how much I fought to return to the path from which I was diverted, every blind turn promising that just ahead lay that idealized road for which I hoped, my unintended path taught me more about myself, others and life in general than I likely would have learned during the existence I imagined at twenty-four. I will finally admit to myself, after seven years of denial, that I am better for having never been able to return.

It is now time that I serve as a better steward for the life I built. There will come a day, in the very distant future, I hope, when it will no longer be mine, and it can belong solely to everyone else through anecdotes passed between acquaintances, if they so choose—the very place from which I so frequently borrowed to piece together this story. But what I have written, my past as I now know it, with all of its missing memories, with all of its editorial pieces provided by me and others, is still mine.

I am the guy who was on law review. I am the guy who was lazy and entitled and who coasted through life. I am the guy who suffered a traumatic brain injury. I am the guy who fought his way out of a hospital bed and back into mainstream society. I am the guy who spent virtually every day trembling at the prospect of failure. I am the guy who was the All-State tennis player. That is my name on the plaque. It is me. I am present. Please note it for the roll. This future, once viewed hopefully as a rapid recovery, now fraught with uncertainty, plagued by a fatigue that will never be fully vanquished and limitations which neither I nor any doctor can precisely identify, is mine.

The doubts will never fully be silenced, no matter how dearly I wish to hush their whisper. Sitting in front of a computer, without anyone to supervise me, I know that no one remains who has the authority to tell me I'm not what I think I am, my "abilities" and my "accomplishments" always left unchallenged by an unconscious mind desperate to affirm life paths already chosen. I am still aware that I may have accidentally created a distorted reality by cherry-picking stories from a long narrative and framing my disappointments in terms of effort and attitude rather than insufficient aptitude, all to create a convenient retelling that leads to the conclusion I want to believe—that I will one day partially control my own destiny. I don't think I was this dishonest with myself, but only time will tell.

Regardless, even if the worst-case scenario is true, even if all the firings, all of the unsuccessful relationships, and all of the mental anguish were the direct results of my permanent infirmity rendering my present persona too injured for anything more than simple survival, and I unknowingly used a series of grandiloquent phrases to perpetrate an extravagant fraud on myself, my ability to manipulate this story means something. It would still show exponential improvement over the weak-minded, hospital-bound boy who seven years ago couldn't breathe without assistance. Even without the ability today to dismiss the most jaded of views, I know that I am still strong enough.

I am tired of mourning the future that never happened, and though I know the stories I heard were about me, I am no longer content to coast into what I believe is mediocrity while talking about my past. I will never fully know who I was, but I have begun to suspect most other people don't know this about themselves, either, and I no longer look for a job or a girlfriend to tell me who I am. I already know enough to stand on my own and believe in me today.

I want to tackle new challenges, I want to help new people, I want to become more than I am right now, and I know that these desires are achievable. I care deeply about what my future will look like, and, for that reason, I swear that I will continue to fight, that I will never again waste my life playing dead.

{the detours}

I know I cannot predict or fully control what is to come but, for the first time, I can stand, look out and firmly declare:

I am not scared.

{acknowledgments}

I would like to acknowledge the people who helped make the publication of this book possible. Thank you to Jeff Portnoy whose diligent review of the opening chapters helped jump-start the editing process, Vonda Lee Morton who suffered through grammatical and tense issues for 320 plus pages to make this book readable, and Mary Ruth who helped clarify the language throughout. And I would like to extend a special thank you to my friends Matthew Blackwelder, Mary Cadden, Seth Sabbath, Michael Goldston and Charlotte Nash who agreed to read my initial attempts to assemble this story, then fought through the text, alerting me to issues and then, in the most supportive way imaginable, offered their suggestions as to how to fix the problems that they saw. I also know that this book would never have been published in its present form without the introductions made during writing groups and the patient efforts of my fellow writers over Saturday morning coffee and without Bob, Jan, and Mark Babcock, who chose to take a chance on me and make my story's publication a reality.

I wanted to extend a final thank you to everyone who has played a role in my recovery, especially those individuals who were close to me during the process, though the list is too long to even begin, and I do not wish to violate anyone's anonymity through an attempted gesture of goodwill. Standing with me or being involved even peripherally in my life at any point during this time was undoubtedly more difficult than it should have been, and I appreciate everyone's contributions and know that my future would look much bleaker were it not for your help along the way.

{resources}

Though suffering a traumatic brain injury can be an incredibly isolating experience, there are a growing number of resources available to aid in the recovery process and to assist those who are the caretakers and loved ones of the injured. I have listed a few websites below as a starting point for those seeking more information and assistance. I hope these sites will provide anyone interested in learning more about brain injury, learning to live with a brain injury, or helping someone recover from their injury with helpful information.

There may be setbacks along your road to recovery, but please don't give up. You are not alone.

- BIAA – Brain Injury Association of America – http://www.biausa.org
- Defense and Veterans Brain Injury Center— http://www.dvbic.org
- U.S. Veteran Services – www.va.gov
- Brain Injury Resource Center - http://www.headinjury.com/library.htm
- NINDS – National Institute of Neurological Disorders & Stroke - http://www.ninds.nih.gov/
- BTF – Brain Trauma Foundation – http://ww.braintrauma.org
- NARIC – National Rehabilitation Information Center – http://www.naric.com
- Traumatic Brain Injury Resource Center – http://www.braininjuryresources.org
- The Brain Injury Recovery Network – http://www.tbirecovery.org

- Betty Clooney Foundation – http://www.bcftbi.org
- Transitional Learning Center – www.Tlcrehab.org
- NIH – National Institutes of Health - http://www.nih.gov/

{about the author}

Neil Ligon resides in Atlanta, Georgia. He is the Director of Advocacy for the Emory Chapter of the Brain Injury Association of Georgia, sits on the Support Group Liaison Committee for the Brain Injury Association of Georgia, and serves as a peer visitor for the Brain Injury Peer Visitor Association. Through these endeavors, he hopes to provide others who have suffered a brain injury and their caretakers with access to the resources available to help them in their recovery, while working to provide anyone interested with the information to better understand these complex injuries.